The Illustrated
ART of MANLINESS

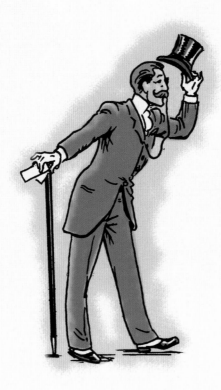

The Illustrated
ART of MANLINESS

The Essential How-To Guide

Survival • Chivalry • Self-Defense
Style • Car Repair • and More!

Brett McKay *and* **The Art of Manliness**

Illustrations by **Ted Slampyak**

LITTLE, BROWN AND COMPANY

New York | Boston | London

Little, Brown and Company
Hachette Book Group
1290 Avenue of the Americas, New York, NY 10104
littlebrown.com

First Edition: May 2017

Little, Brown and Company is a division of Hachette Book Group, Inc.
The Little, Brown name and logo are trademarks of Hachette Book Group, Inc.

The publisher is not responsible for websites (or their content) that are not owned by the publisher.

The Hachette Speakers Bureau provides a wide range of authors for speaking events. To find out more, go to hachettespeakersbureau.com or call (866) 376-6591.

Illustrations by Ted Slampyak

Design by Paul Kepple & Max Vandenberg at Headcase Design

ISBN 978-0-316-36265-8
Library of Congress Control Number: 2017933607

10 9 8 7 6 5 4 3 2

Q-MA

Printed in the United States of America

For Men

If you can keep your head when all about you
Are losing theirs and blaming it on you,

If you can trust yourself when all men doubt you,
But make allowance for their doubting too;

If you can wait and not be tired by waiting,
Or being lied about, don't deal in lies,

Or being hated, don't give way to hating,
And yet don't look too good, nor talk too wise:

....

If you can dream—and not make dreams your master;
If you can think—and not make thoughts your aim;

If you can meet with Triumph and Disaster
And treat those two impostors just the same;

If you can bear to hear the truth you've spoken
Twisted by knaves to make a trap for fools,

Or watch the things you gave your life to, broken,
And stoop and build 'em up with worn-out tools:

....

If you can make one heap of all your winnings
And risk it on one turn of pitch-and-toss,

And lose, and start again at your beginnings
And never breathe a word about your loss;

If you can force your heart and nerve and sinew
To serve your turn long after they are gone,

And so hold on when there is nothing in you
Except the Will which says to them "Hold on!"

....

If you can talk with crowds and keep your virtue,
Or walk with Kings—nor lose the common touch,

If neither foes nor loving friends can hurt you,
If all men count with you, but none too much;

If you can fill the unforgiving minute
With sixty seconds' worth of distance run,

Yours is the Earth and everything that's in it,
And—which is more—you'll be a Man, my son!

IF—

Rudyard Kipling (1910)

CONTENTS

Introduction

Chapter One: The ADVENTURER

Chapter Two: The GENTLEMAN

Chapter Three: The TECHNICIAN

Chapter Four: The WARRIOR

Chapter Five: The FAMILY MAN

Chapter Six: The LEADER

INTRODUCTION

What Makes a Man?

MANHOOD HAS always been about the competence to be effective in the world. To be a man means to be skilled in the range of tasks that are critical to survive and thrive in society—becoming both physically proficient and culturally competent. To be manly means acquiring a breadth of skills so that you can deftly and adroitly handle any situation you find yourself in.

The French idea of savoir faire (pronounced "sahv-wah fair") encapsulates this notion. You already know what it is: James Bond embodies it. Teddy Roosevelt had it in spades, and so did many of our grandfathers (I know mine did). Men with savoir faire can change a flat tire, dress sharp for any event, converse with both truck drivers and diplomats, and immobilize an armed attacker. Developing savoir faire means becoming a Renaissance man: smooth, smart, handy, and resourceful.

Across cultures, research shows that the traits women find most attractive in men are competence and effectiveness—not sports cars or six-pack abs. (Napoleon Dynamite was right: Chicks dig guys with skills.) These traits are prerequisites for the independence and autonomy that cultures across the world expect from men. They enable us to live satisfying, self-directed lives.

Plus, it simply feels awesome to know you possess the skills and confidence to walk into any situation and know how to act, how to own the room, and how to solve any problem that arises. Nietzsche said it best: "Happiness is the feeling of power increasing." As you expand your skill set, you increase your ability to be effective in the world around you. You become more powerful, more potent, and that feels good.

I started The Art of Manliness in 2008 to help men develop savoir faire in a world that has left many men adrift, lacking the confidence, focus, skills, and virtues that the men we look up to embodied. This book fills that void—helping you perfect the skills to be honorable, well-rounded, capable husbands, fathers, brothers, and citizens.

BUT WHAT SKILLS DOES A MODERN MAN NEED TO KNOW?

It's a debate that has gone on for centuries among men and will probably continue for centuries more. With *The Illustrated Art of Manliness*, we add our contribution to this great conversation. While we don't cover every conceivable skill a man needs to know, we think this volume represents a very good start. We wed the best of the past to the best of the present, offering guidance for a multidimensional, flourishing life.

We've divided the book into six chapters that correspond to the roles that most men assume at one time or another in contemporary life: adventurer, gentleman, technician, warrior, family man, and leader. Among them you'll find a nice mix of "hard" and "soft" skills that together build a constellation of all-around capability. For most of us living in capitalist, democratic societies, soft skills like dressing well, leading effectively, and displaying charisma help us excel. But we still need hard skills, like knowing how to fight or start a fire, even though we no longer need to survive in the wild or constantly guard against physical threats. Whether you're striving for the corner office or find yourself lost in the woods, it's better to have these skills and not need them than it is to need them, and not have them.

We may not be arctic explorers, race-car drivers, survivalists, or doctors—but we can learn from them. For each skill, we've done the research and consulted with top practitioners in relevant fields to deliver the advice ahead. Nevertheless, use your own good judgment, be responsible for your own safety, and be respectful of others.

We hope this book inspires you to grow and challenge yourself by learning new skills. You'll increase your competence, your effectiveness, and your usefulness. And based on thousands of years of human history, not to mention the feeling you get when your skills match the scenario, that's pretty damn manly.

—Brett McKay, *founder*, The Art of Manliness

Chapter 1

The ADVENTURER

An inconvenience is only an adventure wrongly considered;
an adventure is an inconvenience rightly considered.

—G. K. Chesterton

SOMETHING IN the masculine heart calls men to explore the unknown. Such adventure requires seizing possibilities, and you don't know what all of them will be before setting out. There's risk in the endeavor. There's a chance you'll fail. It's a chance to test your mettle—an opportunity to "shew yourself a man," as the Bible puts it. Through adventure, a man has a chance to take risks, improvise, and show deftness of skill in an unfamiliar environment. He has an opportunity to turn *if* into *did*.

Even today, in a world that has been mapped precisely, adventure is still available for the man who really wants it, and is of the mind to find it wherever he goes. Jack London considered all of life to be an "adventure path," and this chapter will provide the skills you'll need for your journey.

FELL A TREE

Whether you're cutting down a tree for firewood, a better view of the lake, or as a guarantee to never rake leaves again, there are few things more fun—or more dangerous—than watching it fall while yelling "Timber!" at the top of your lungs. The same angle-cutting technique applies for both chainsaws and felling axes.

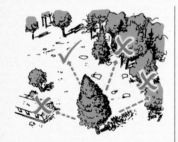 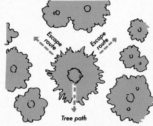 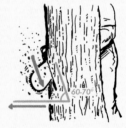

1: DETERMINE where the tree should fall. Look for areas that are downhill and clear of any structures or other trees.

2: PLAN two escape routes opposite where the tree will fall. They should be about 45 degrees apart. Clear any branches or obstacles from these paths.

3: MAKE your initial, or notch, cut at the base of the fall side of the tree. Cut at a 60–70 degree angle to about one-third through the tree's diameter.

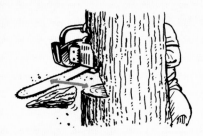

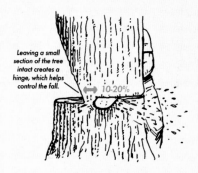

4: TO finish the notch cut, cut a line parallel to where the first cut ended, and remove the wedge.

5: MAKE your final, or felling, cut on the opposite side of the tree, a few inches above the previous parallel cut. Stop when 10–20% of the trunk remains.

Leaving a small section of the trunk intact creates a hinge to help control the fall.

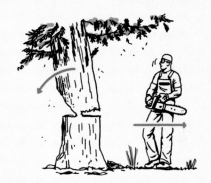

6: AS the tree falls, quickly but carefully back away along your escape route.

SPLIT FIREWOOD

Henry Ford famously said, "Chop your own wood and it will warm your twice." For most men, "chopping" wood means grabbing an ax and hacking away with no real thought. You're not most men, though. You know that splitting wood in the most effective and efficient way means using the right tools and the correct form. Familiarize yourself with both and you'll resemble Paul Bunyan in no time.

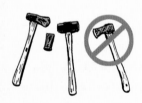

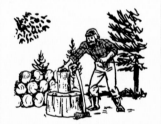

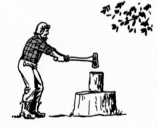

1: GATHER the right tools. Use a splitting maul instead of an ax, or consider a sledgehammer and a wedge for green wood or larger pieces.

2: PLACE the log on a sturdy surface like a chopping block, or on the ground.

3: AIM for preexisting hairline cracks in the wood, where it splits easiest. Stand so that the maul head meets the log when your arms are extended.

Ax heads get stuck while mauls split and separate the wood.

Driving your maul head into rocky ground will dull the blade.

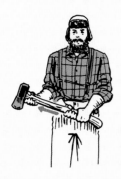

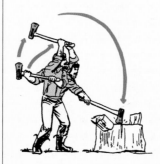

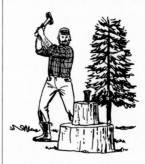

4: GRIP the maul handle like a baseball bat and then slide your hands far apart, holding the maul across your body.

5: BRING the maul head behind your body, leading with your top hand. Keep the momentum going as you slide your hands together and bring the maul over your head, extending your arms to maximize the force of your swing.

6: FOR larger pieces, first create a cut with your maul. Insert a wedge into the cut, and then drive it through with a sledgehammer.

START A FIRE WITHOUT MATCHES

Food, water, fire, and shelter are critical to your survival in an emergency situation. Fire provides warmth and protection, offers up a signal, cooks food and sterilizes water, and offers comfort. Carrying a bit of dry tinder, matches, a lighter, or a flint and steel setup will ensure you're never without a roaring fire, but you can still spawn a spark if you lack those easy resources.

HAND DRILL

1: CUT a notch into the side of a flat piece of wood approximately the width of your finger to make a friction board. Carve the end of a perfectly straight stick to fit the notch and make a spindle. The notch and spindle should seat perfectly together.

2: PLACE a tinder bundle beneath the notch.

3: PLACE the spindle in the notch and pinch the top of the spindle with your open palms.

4: MOVING your palms back and forth, rotate the spindle in the notch. Maintain constant downward pressure.

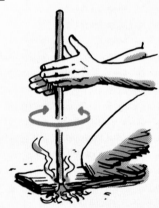

5: WORK the spindle as fast as possible until smoke begins to form in the notch and an ember falls into the tinder bundle. It may take several minutes for this to happen.

There was the fire, snapping and crackling and promising life with every dancing flame.

—Jack London, "To Build a Fire"

BOW DRILL

1: START with the hand drill setup: a friction board, spindle, and tinder bundle.

2: FIND a curved, bow-shaped stick the length of your arm.

3: TIE a string to one end of the bow, wrap the string around your spindle, pull it tight, and attach it to the other end of the bow.

4: FIND a concave rock or piece of hardwood with a depression in the center to act as a bearing block.

5: PUT your weight on the bearing block while holding the friction plate in place with your foot.

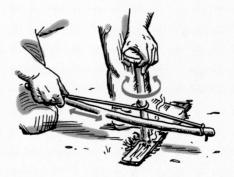

6: DRAW the bow back and forth as fast as possible, using a sawing motion, while maintaining control to force the spindle to rotate until an ember is formed.

BATTERY

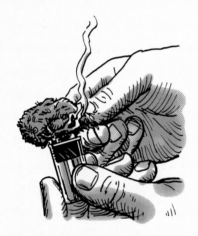

CROSS the positive and negative ends of a battery with steel wool to ignite it.

LENS REFRACTION

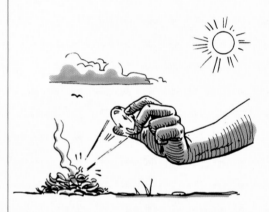

TILT a lens in direct sunlight to focus a small, concentrated beam on the center of a tinder bundle, holding it in place until it ignites.

BUILD A ROARING CAMPFIRE

Few things are more primitively satisfying than taking wood to flame in the great outdoors. To make a rip-roaring, s'mores-toasting, butt-warming fire that will be the envy of the campsite, start with dry tinder and keep it going with plenty of well-seasoned wood.

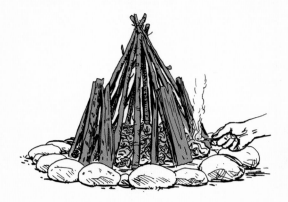

1: SELECT a site away from trees, shrubs, and other greenery. Clear the area of grass, leaves, and other flammable material.

2: FORM a rock circle with a 2- to 3-foot diameter around where you want to build a fire.

3: USE dry, flammable tinder like crumpled paper, leaves, or bark as the base.

4: PLACE thin wood shavings on top of the tinder.

5: CROSS pencil-thick twigs over the tinder and wood shavings pile, leaving room in between for air circulation.

6: IGNITE using a match or lighter. Once it starts, blow on the fire to increase oxygen and heat so the wood catches quickly.

7: ADD larger pieces of kindling and then full logs as needed to keep the flames going.

SURVIVE FALLING THROUGH ICE

While no ice is guaranteed to be safe to walk on, the rule of thumb is that you shouldn't venture out onto clear ice that is less than 2 inches thick; a safer bet is 4 inches. "Snow ice," or white ice, will need to be at least 8 inches thick to support you. When walking on ice, carry rescue ice picks with you. They're cheap and can make a life-or-death difference. You can also make your own with a couple nails and dowels.

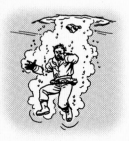 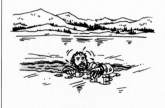 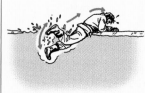

1: DO not breathe in the water. Your body's shock response will cause you to gasp and hyperventilate. Resist this force. The shock will wear off in one to three minutes—and you have fifteen to forty-five minutes before you lose consciousness. Try to stay calm.

2: ORIENT yourself and get back to where you fell through. This ice held you before, so it should be sturdy enough to help you crawl out.

3: DON'T pull yourself straight up. Get horizontal, and kick your feet while using your elbows for traction to get up out of the water and onto the ice. Pull and kick until you're out.

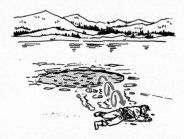

4: LIE flat on ice and roll away—don't stand up. This reduces the risk of further cracking the ice. Find warm, dry shelter immediately.

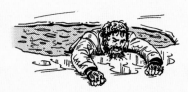

5: IF you can't get out, stop thrashing to conserve heat and energy. Put your arms on the ice and don't move them—they may freeze to the ice, keeping you from slipping into the water if you lose consciousness and giving rescuers more time to reach you. Get as much of your body onto the ice as you can—water draws heat from the body twenty-five times faster than air.

Your beard can also freeze on the ice and save you.

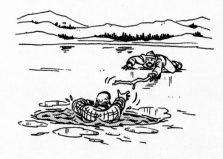

6: IF your friend falls through, call 911 and coach them through this process. Don't go out to them on the hazardous ice—two victims are worse than one. If they can't get out on their own, extend a looped rope they can put around their arms, or a tree branch or ladder to hold on to.

SURVIVE A BEAR ATTACK

Bear attacks are rare, but you should always be prepared while camping or hiking in the wild. How you handle an attack depends on the type of bear you encounter.

GRIZZLY BEAR

How to Identify a Grizzly (Brown) Bear

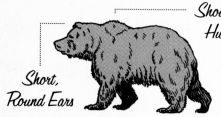

Shoulder Hump

Short, Round Ears

- 6.5 feet long
- 400–800 pounds
- Found in Europe, Asia, Canada, and U.S. Pacific Northwest

Always Carry Bear Spray

STAY PREPARED

1: ALWAYS carry bear spray.

2: IF you suspect bears in the area, make noise. Sing, talk to yourself, etc.

3: NEVER leave food on the trail. Always pick up all trash, even organic.

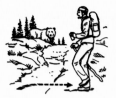

ENCOUNTERING A GRIZZLY

WALK AWAY slowly; don't run. Be prepared to spray bear at a distance of around 25 feet. Be as non-threatening as possible: make yourself smaller and avoid eye contact.

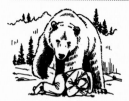

IF CHARGED

DON'T RUN. Lie on the ground and play dead; protect your head and stomach. Wait ten to twenty minutes after the bear leaves to get up.

BLACK BEAR

How to Identify a Black Bear

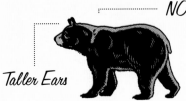

NO Shoulder Hump

Taller Ears

- 5 feet long
- 100–300 pounds
- Black bears aren't always black; they are often brown or cinnamon colored. Common throughout North America and East Asia.

I Repeat, Always Carry Bear Spray

STAY PREPARED

1: ALWAYS carry bear spray.

2: IF you suspect bears in the area, make noise. Sing, talk to yourself, etc.

3: NEVER leave food on the trail. Always pick up all trash, even organic.

4: ADD bells to your pack.

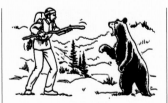

ENCOUNTERING A BLACK BEAR

DON'T RUN; stand your ground and make yourself look as big as possible. Shout, wave your arms, and create a commotion. Never try to climb a tree.

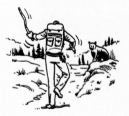

IF CHARGED

FIGHT BACK. Aim for the nose or other sensitive areas. Use rocks/sticks if available. Let the bear be the first to run.

MAKE A TORCH LIKE INDIANA JONES

Whether you're navigating the woods in a survival situation or hunting for treasure deep in the tunnels of an ancient temple, all it takes to make a torch are a few common supplies.

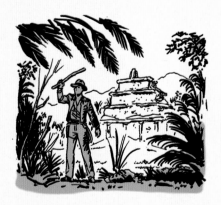

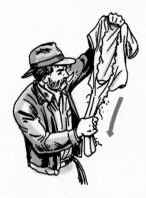

1: FIND a green branch or stick. You'll need a one at least 2 feet long and a few inches thick. The greener the better—you don't want your handle to burn along with the flame.

2: IF using man-made fuels, cut a strip of cotton cloth about 1 foot wide, and 2–3 feet long. The longer you need your torch to burn, the bigger to cut the cloth. For fuel, you can use natural (tree pitch/resin, bark) or man-made (kerosene, gas, lighter fluid) materials. If using natural fuels, forgo the cloth and cover the end of the stick with the bark or pitch, and skip to Step 6.

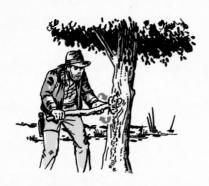

3: WRAP the cloth around the end of the stick so it creates a bulge in the cloth.

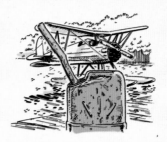

5: SOAK the cloth in fuel for a few minutes before lighting. Dry cloth will char and burn away.

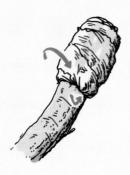

4: TUCK in the end.

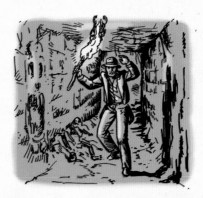

6: LIGHT your torch! If using natural fuels, it may take 30–60 seconds to get lit. Be especially cautious in dry, wooded areas. Your new torch should last 20–50 minutes.

JUMP FROM A SPEEDING CAR

It's a classic Hollywood scenario: the bad guys cut the brake lines, the good guys get in the car, and chaos ensues. But while you're unlikely to be the target of such a villainous act, brakes do sometimes fail. If you find yourself in a runaway car with no way to slow down, your best bet might be to bail.

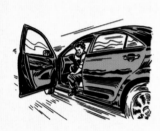 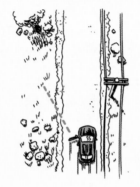 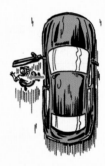

1: OPEN the door as wide as possible to lower your chances of getting caught on the car when you jump.

2: LOOK ahead for a landing spot that's soft (like patches of grass and dirt) and free of obstacles like rocks or road signs.

3: JUMP at an angle perpendicular to the car's movement so you minimize the chance of rolling back toward the road when you land.

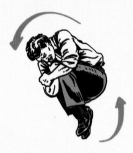

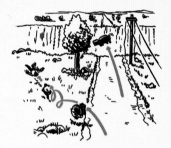

4: TUCK yourself into a ball, lowering your head and bringing your arms and legs in tight to your body.

5: ROLL when you land to spread the impact out as much as possible.

Try to land on your shoulder to reduce injuries to more vital parts of your body.

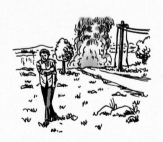

6: GET away from the roadside to avoid getting run over by passing vehicles. Evaluate any injuries you might have and get checked out by paramedics ASAP.

ESCAPE A SINKING CAR

More than 10,000 water immersion auto accidents happen each year. Nearly 12% of American bridges have been deemed "structurally deficient" by the Federal Highway Administration. It's scary to think that one might collapse while you're driving over it—and it's highly unlikely. But a bridge collapse is hardly the only way to end up in a submerged vehicle. Many drivers simply skid out around a curve, go over a guardrail, and end up in a body of water.

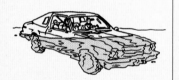 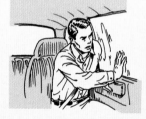 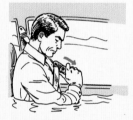

1: STAY calm. On average, you'll have 30–120 seconds of float time before the car sinks. That's plenty of time to escape.

2: DON'T open the door. It's possible to escape this way, but difficult to do even in just a foot of water. The car will also sink almost immediately after, making it impossible for passengers to escape.

3: REMEMBER four simple steps: "Seat belts. Children. Windows. Out." First, unbuckle your seat belt. If the buckle is stuck, cut it off.

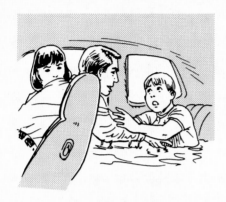

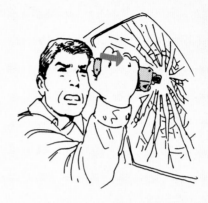

4: MAKE sure children and passengers can get out of their seat belts. Guide and instruct them to exit through their own window if possible, or pull them to the front of the car.

5: ESCAPE through window. Try rolling it down first. If that doesn't work, use an auto rescue tool or the prongs of your headrest to safely shatter the window. It's nearly impossible to break using your arms or legs.

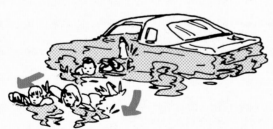

Swim out through the window to safety.

JUMP FROM A BRIDGE INTO WATER

Few things are more dangerous than diving into an unknown body of water from a high place. Professional cliff divers do underwater surveys before attempting a dive from any height, and for good cause—from a height of 20 feet, your body will be traveling at 25 miles per hour when it hits the water. Do not attempt this for fun. But if you're forced to leap from a bridge in extreme circumstances, you give yourself the chance to survive injury or death.

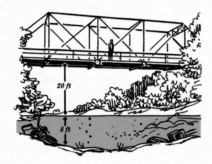

1: IDEALLY, make sure the water is deep enough. Aim for the darkest part of the water for a visual cue. From a height of 20 feet, the water should be at least 8 feet deep. Add 2 feet of water depth for every additional 10 feet of jump height. Although some professional cliff divers can enter the water safely from more than 100 feet, all jumps risk serious injury or death.

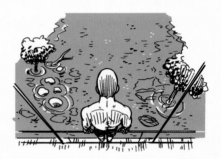

2: PICK a landing spot free of underwater obstacles like tree roots and rocks.

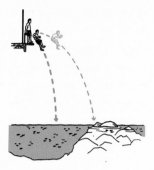

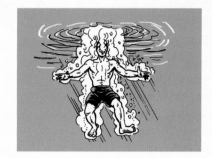

3: TAKE a large step off the bridge. Avoid jumping, which can alter your trajectory.

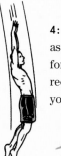

4: ARCH your back slightly as you fall to avoid rotating forward, and raise your arms directly above your head to form your body into a pencil shape.

Pencil dives minimize surface area and reduce impact on your body.

5: SPREAD your arms and legs out once you enter the water to slow your body down.

6: SWIM to the surface and find a place to climb out.

SWIM AT a 90-degree angle to the current to avoid getting swept downstream.

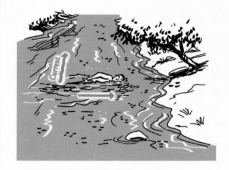

FIND WATER IN THE WILD

Survival experts refer to the Rule of Threes: the average person can go three minutes without air, three hours without shelter (in a harsh environment), three days without water, and three weeks without food. If you're breathing and have shelter, your next step should be to find a water source. With a little ingenuity, water may not be far away—but remember, any water you find in the wild should be boiled or treated to kill pathogens.

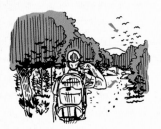 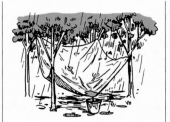 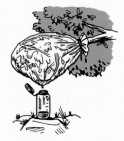

1: LOOK for readily available water by following the direction of animal tracks and flocks of birds, and by listening for the sound of rushing water.

2: COLLECT water by hanging a tarp to catch rain, channeled into a container.

3: HARVEST water from plants by securing a plastic bag around the foliage, letting the plant's transpiration collect at the bottom of the bag.

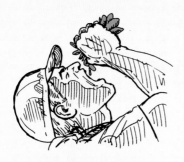

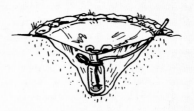

4: SQUEEZE water out of succulents like cactus and moss.

5: MAKE an underground still by digging a hole with a container at the center. Cover with plastic, make the edges air tight, and weigh down the center with a rock. Wait for the ground moisture to gather and run down the plastic into the container.

Run a tube from the container to the outside of the well so you can take drinks without removing the plastic.

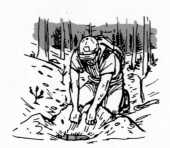

6: DIG a well to locate groundwater near low spots in the terrain, on beaches, or next to dry river or creek beds.

LAND A PLANE

Pilots spend thousands of hours learning to operate the wall of controls in modern cockpits. While autopilot systems make the majority of airtime downright mundane, landing a plane still requires a manual touch. If the pilot of your next flight is incapacitated, it may be up to you to take over.

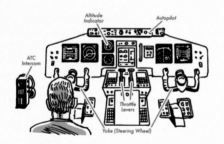

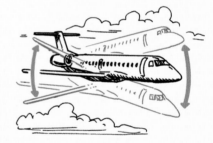

1: IDENTIFY the main controls and instruments. Pull back on the throttle to reduce speed, push forward to increase. Pull back on the yoke to increase altitude, push it forward to descend.

2: ESTABLISH a stable flight position. If the autopilot is on, leave it on. If the plane is in a turn, ascending, or descending, use the yoke and throttle to level the plane and reach a stable speed (~500 knots).

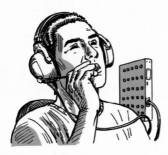

3: CALL ATC (Air Traffic Control) using the intercom to the left of the yoke. Say "Mayday," identify your flight number, and describe the situation.

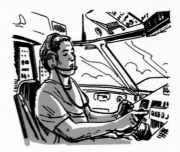

4: FOLLOW ATC's guidance to adjust your speed, direction, and altitude to get lined up with the nearest runway. Deploy the landing gear as you're making your final approach.

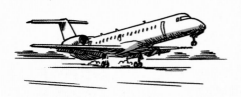

5: PULL up on the yoke and pull back on the throttle just before you land to decrease speed and raise the nose of the plane.

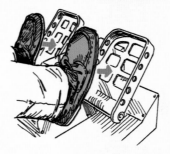

6: DEPRESS the pedals at your feet to engage the wheel brakes and stop the plane.

SURVIVE A PLANE CRASH

We think of plane crashes as catastrophic, unsurvivable events. Thankfully, that isn't the case—the National Transportation Safety Board found that the survival rate of crashes is 95.7%. Take note of another tidbit the FAA and NTSB uncovered: 40% of airplane crash fatalities might have been prevented had passengers taken proper action.

The odds of being in a plane crash are slim, but they're not zero.
Here's how to increase your chance of walking away.

NINETY SECONDS TO GET OUT

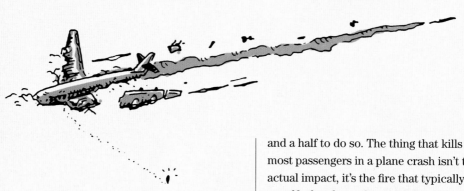

IF YOU'VE survived the crash landing, you have a good chance of getting out of the airplane alive. But you only have a minute and a half to do so. The thing that kills most passengers in a plane crash isn't the actual impact, it's the fire that typically engulfs the plane afterward. It takes, on average, just ninety seconds for a fire to burn through the plane's fuselage and consume everything in it. If that sounds scary, it should. Get out of the plane!

THE FIVE ROW RULE

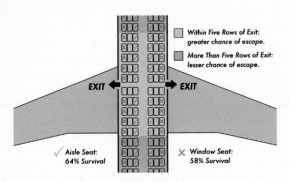

Within Five Rows of Exit: greater chance of escape.

More Than Five Rows of Exit: lesser chance of escape.

EXIT

EXIT

✓ Aisle Seat: 64% Survival

✗ Window Seat: 58% Survival

STATISTICS ARE inconclusive about whether the front or the rear of the plane is safer in a crash. Every plane crash is different, so focus on finding a seat near an exit. Crash survivors typically only have to move an average of five rows to escape. The best seat to have is in the exit row. If you can't snag that seat, go for the aisle. You'll increase your chance of survival by 6% over a window seat.

MAKE AN ACTION PLAN

OUR BRAINS react slowly to disaster. Instead of springing to action when something unexpected happens, our brain shrugs and assumes that what is going on can't be so bad, because truly bad events are so out of the ordinary.

TO OVERCOME this "normalcy bias," make an action plan as soon as you sit down. Read the safety card. Spot the nearest exit and count the rows to it. Size up the passengers around you and look for obsta-

cles to your exit. If traveling with kids and another adult, discuss who will be responsible for whom in the event of an accident. Mentally rehearse springing to action as soon as the plane comes to a stop.

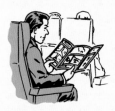

THE PLUS 3/MINUS 8 RULE

CLOSE TO 80% of all plane crashes occur during the first three minutes after takeoff or the final eight minutes before landing.

You don't need to be paranoid —just pay attention.

PUT ON YOUR OXYGEN MASK AS SOON AS IT DROPS

SECURE YOUR mask first before helping others secure theirs. You're useless to others if you're not getting oxygen to your brain.

BRACE YOURSELF

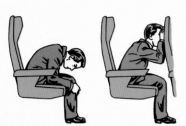

IT MAY seem silly to think that curling up in a ball will help you survive a plane crash, but brace positions work. They reduce the velocity of your head when it slams into the seat in front of you, and minimizes limb flailing.

MAKE SURE your seat belt is securely fastened—low and tight. Those bad boys are designed to withstand 3,000 pounds of force, or about three times as much as you can handle before passing out.

USE YOUR CELL PHONE AS A SURVIVAL TOOL

A cell phone is the single most useful survival tool you have…as long as you have service and plenty of battery power. Once it dies, your device might seem as useful as a rock, until you look inside. Crack it open to find tools that might save your life.

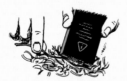

Battery

1: USE a spare wire or piece of steel wool to connect the terminals of the battery together. This short circuit technique can create enough heat or sparks to start a fire.

Mirror

2: NEARLY every phone has a mirror behind the screen. Use it to signal search-and-rescue teams or to reflect sunlight onto a tinder pile to create a spot hot enough to catch flame.

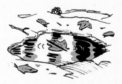

Speaker

3: SPEAKERS typically have magnets you can use with a needle to create a compass. Wipe the needle several times against the magnet in the same direction, and then place the needle on a leaf floating in a calm pool of water. The needle will point due north.

Circuit Board

4: SHARPEN hard circuit boards on rocks to create knives, arrowheads, and fishing lures.

PADDLE A CANOE

Paddling a canoe may seem as straightforward as peeling an orange, but subtle motions differentiate an efficient stroke from a poor one. Splashing and zig-zagging around lakes and rivers is the stuff of mere boys. You should canoe like a man: calmly, confidently, quickly moving toward your next adventure.

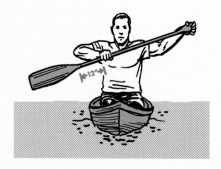

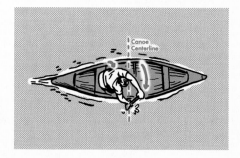

1: GRIP the paddle with your right hand a foot above the blade and your left hand on the grip at the top.

2: REACH forward, slightly twisting your torso to put the paddle into the water at the centerline, or middle, of the canoe's body.

For paddling on the port (left) side of the canoe, use the opposite grip.

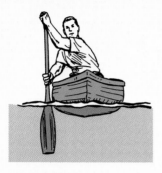

3: PUT the paddle into the water vertically, keeping the blade's face perpendicular to the canoe. The paddle should be deep enough that its contour matches that of the canoe's hull.

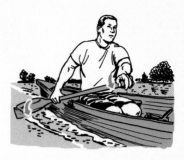

5: HALFWAY through your stroke, gently rotate the blade to be parallel to the boat by turning your grip hand so its back points away from you.

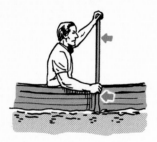

4: DRAW the paddle toward you through the water, keeping the blade perpendicular to the canoe as you use your shoulders and torso to pull, rather than just your arms.

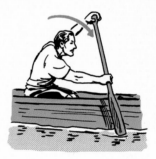

6: PULL the paddle out of the water with minimal splashing and stretch forward to start the process over, keeping the blade close to the water to minimize excess movement.

BUILD A LOG RAFT

Huck Finn meandered down the Mississippi in a raft, and the explorer Thor Heyerdahl crossed the Pacific in one he called Kon-Tiki. Try to use lighter-weight woods like balsa, pine, or oak, and make your knots as tight as possible to avoid shifting once you're underway.

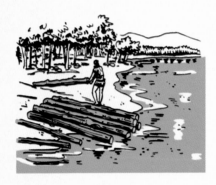

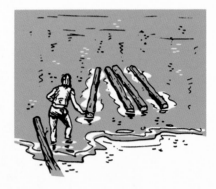

1: GATHER six to eight 10-foot logs at least 10 inches in diameter, and four thinner 10-foot logs at least 6 inches in diameter.

2: DRAG the logs into shallow water and arrange the thicker ones next to each other to make a platform.

Assemble the raft in the water to make it easier to move.

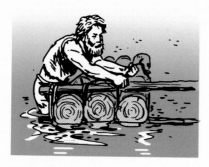

3: SANDWICH the larger logs with two thin logs and use rope or thick vines to tie them in place.

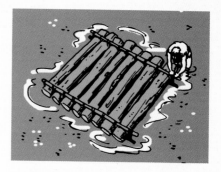

5: REPEAT on the other side, using the last two thin logs to secure the other side of the raft.

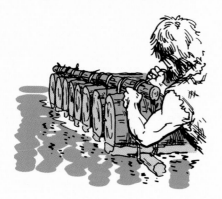

4: CONTINUE to secure each larger log in place. The thin logs will pinch the platform, and hold it in place.

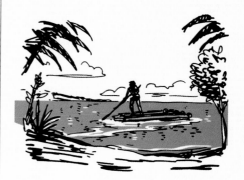

6: USE a long branch as an oar.

SURVIVE A TORNADO

Tornadoes can occur without warning any time of day, even if there isn't a thunderstorm in the area. Most occur in the afternoon and are preceded by telltale conditions:

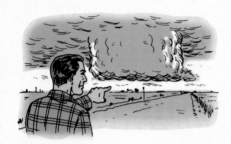

- A pea-soup green sky and/or a low, dark cloud.
- Strong, persistent rotation in the cloud base.
- Whirling dust on the ground under a cloud base—tornadoes sometimes have no funnel!
- Hail or heavy rain followed by dead calm or a fast, intense wind shift.
- A loud, continuous roar or rumble that doesn't fade in a few seconds like thunder.
- Small, bright flashes at ground level near a thunderstorm. These indicate power lines being snapped by wind.

TAKE COVER

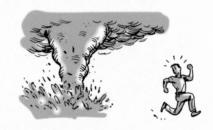

ONCE THERE'S an official tornado warning—or if you see the above signs—seek shelter immediately. A tornado's biggest danger is flying debris. It can turn two-by-fours, bricks, and branches into deadly missiles.

HERE'S HOW TO SURVIVE

1: IN a house. If you don't have a dedicated storm shelter, take cover in the basement, or failing that, an interior bathroom, hallway, or closet without windows on the lowest floor. The more walls between you and the wind, the better. Don't position yourself under a large, heavy object that's on the

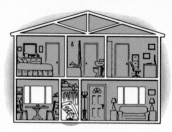

floor(s) above you—like a piano or refrigerator. It could come crashing down. Cover yourself with a mattress or blankets, or crawl under a sturdy table or workbench. Do not open the windows of the house.

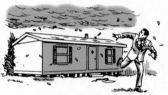

2: IN a mobile home. Get out! You're fifteen times more likely to die there than in any other location.

3: AT a store or office. Take shelter in an interior room or bathroom on the ground

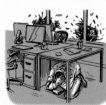

floor — one that's free of or far from windows. Crouch facedown and cover your head with your hands and arms.

Interior stairwells are also good spots. Avoid elevators.

4: "LONG-SPAN" buildings (shopping malls, big box stores, theaters, and gyms) can be particularly dangerous places to be during a tornado, as the roof is often only supported by the exterior walls. Look for a windowless bathroom or storage room on the lowest level. Hunker down under something that might provide stronger support, like a door frame, or under something sturdy, like theater seats.

5: ON the road. Your car is one of the most dangerous places you can be when a tornado strikes. Get inside

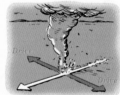

a building, or head for a ditch. Do not take shelter under an overpass or bridge.

6: OUTSIDE. If there are no shelters around, lie flat in a low area of ground like a ditch and cover your head with

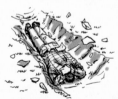

your arms. Pick a spot away from trees and other potential projectiles.

PERFORM THE FIREMAN'S CARRY

Carrying another person is hard, especially when they're unresponsive. Heavy heads, limp limbs, and asymmetrical weight distribution will have even the strongest of heroes struggling to move someone. If you need to pick someone up and carry them away from danger, use the same methods as the pros.

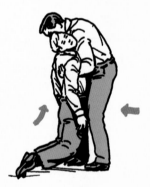

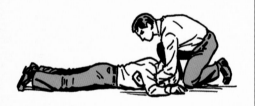

1: TAKE a knee and pull the person toward you, gripping under their arms.

2: PULL the person into a standing position so that they are facing toward you. Lift with your legs instead of your back.

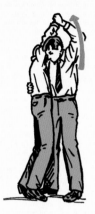

3: GRAB their wrist and swing their arm over your head and around your neck.

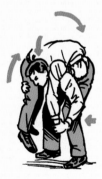

4: BEND your knees, put your free arm between their legs, and let their upper body slump onto your shoulders and back.

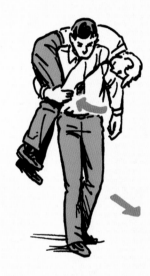

5: TRANSFER their wrist to the arm threaded between their legs and start carrying them to safety.

MAKE URBAN SURVIVAL CANDLES

Whether it's a well-thought-out bug-out bag or a basic kit for when the power goes out, a collection of gear including food, water, lights, and first-aid materials is always a good thing to have on hand. But if you find yourself in a situation without a source of light, you may have alternative options with these homemade candles. All you need is a fuel source and a wick.

Be Prepared!

—Boy Scout Motto

ALMOST ANY natural fiber will act as a wick and almost any oil or fat will act as a fuel. Submerge the wick in your fuel source, leaving a small portion of it exposed so it can be lit. Coat the exposed tip with fuel before lighting to promote the movement of fuel up the wick.

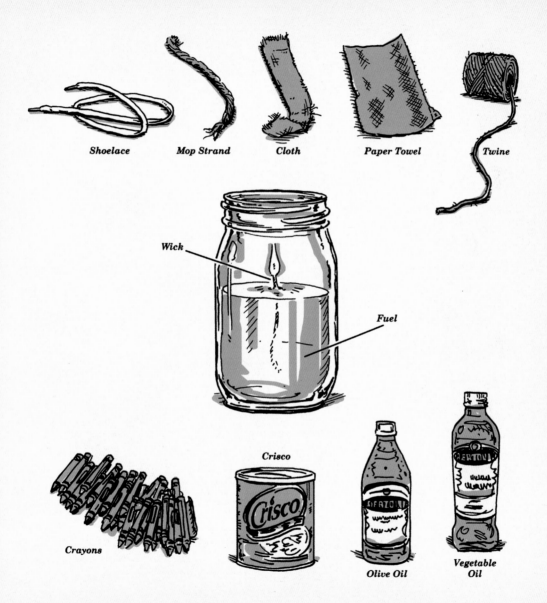

Shoelace **Mop Strand** **Cloth** **Paper Towel** **Twine**

Wick

Fuel

Crayons **Crisco** **Olive Oil** **Vegetable Oil**

Chapter 2

The
GENTLEMAN

Courtesy is as much a mark of a gentleman as courage.

—Theodore Roosevelt

THE ANCIENT Greeks called their gentlemen *kalos kagathos,* and required that they be well-groomed and well-dressed, take part in cultured discussion, and exhibit an even temper, physical strength, and bravery. In 9th-century BC China, the *I Ching* served as a guide for would-be *junzi,* or men who pursued the virtue of *ren.* Confucius described such a man as one who "wishing to be established himself, seeks also to establish others; wishing to be enlarged himself, he seeks also to enlarge others."

Today, a gentleman cares about how he looks and how he behaves. Put simply, he gives a damn. He strives for polish not out of vanity, but out of a concern for other people. His presence adds to the ambiance and texture of an occasion. When he practices courtesy, he uplifts those with whom he interacts.

Gentlemanliness also requires strength underneath the polish. A gentleman's respect is premised on restraint. That he could act as a barbarian, but instead chooses to behave with class, is what gives etiquette its power. As John Wayne declares in *McLintock!,* "You've got to be a man first, before you can be a gentleman."

TIE A FULL WINDSOR NECKTIE KNOT

You're about to go into a big business meeting. Your suit is perfectly fitted, your shoes are shined, your shirt is pressed. Which necktie knot do you go with? It has to make an impression, but not be flashy. It needs to convey power, confidence, and authority. The choice is simple—the full Windsor (also called the Windsor or double Windsor). This knot is often worn for more formal occasions and meetings: weddings, important business meetings, and presidential debates. Because it's a large knot, it should be worn with a spread collar. For men who are stout, or have wider faces and necks, the Windsor will look proportional to your build and mug, and should be your go-to tie knot.

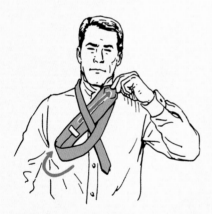

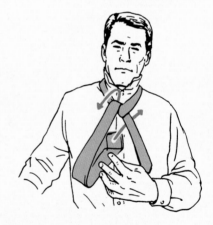

1: DRAPE the tie around your neck. Cross the wide part of the tie over the narrow end, and start to bring it up through the hole between collar and tie.

2: AFTER bringing it up through the hole, pull the wide end down toward the front.

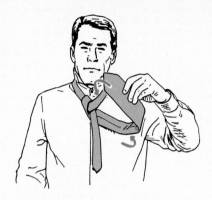

3: BRING the wide end behind the narrow end and to the right. Then pull the wide end back through the loop again.

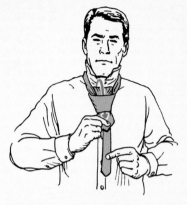

5: BRING the wide end up through the loop a third time, and pull it through the knot in front.

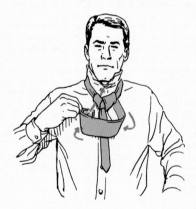

4: WRAP the wide end around the triangle by pulling it from right to left.

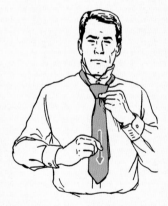

6: TIGHTEN the knot and center it with both hands.

TIE A BOW TIE

START WITH the tie around your neck, allowing the left end (A) to be a little longer than the right end (B). Cross end A over end B.

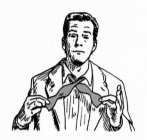

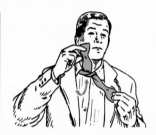

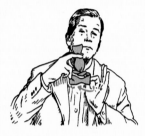

1: TAKE end A and tuck it up in the hole between your neck and tie.

2: FOLD end B at its widest part, holding it sideways. It should look bow-shaped.

3: DROP end A over folded end B. Fold end A up (insert).

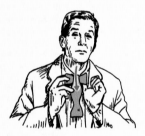

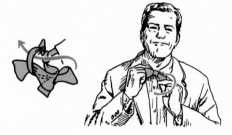

4: THE tricky part: pass folded end A under and behind folded end B on your left and through the loop behind folded end B (insert).

5: TIGHTEN knot by holding both folded ends and pulling carefully. Straighten as needed.

CARRY A HANDKERCHIEF

Handkerchiefs are, well, pretty handy. While women carry a purse stocked with things like tissue packs, most men do not. And yet our noses run just as often. When you carry a hankie, you don't have to scrounge for a tissue to deal with your dripping schnozz, or wipe your nose on your sleeve. And you can mop your brow with it when you're sitting on the front porch drinking mint juleps.

But the best reason to carry a handkerchief has nothing to do with you. It's the chance to lend it to others. Put one in your pocket when you go see a tear-jerker movie with your girlfriend or accompany your wife to a funeral. The offer of a soft hankie is a gallant and chivalrous gesture.

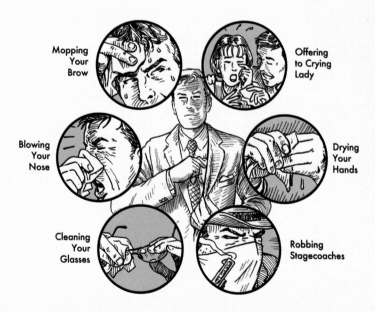

Mopping Your Brow

Offering to Crying Lady

Blowing Your Nose

Drying Your Hands

Cleaning Your Glasses

Robbing Stagecoaches

TIE A SCARF

Scarves are a great way to stay toasty when the winter wind comes biting. Sport any of these styles and you'll be a dapper fellow about town.

The first three ways are for medium-length scarves, and will serve you well in cool temperatures—above freezing and into the 50s. The final two ways are for longer scarves, and are better for those days that dip below the freezing mark.

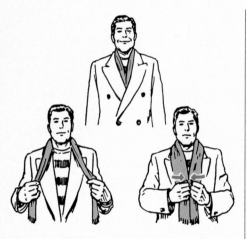

The Drape

SIMPLY DRAPE the scarf around your neck, with equal lengths on both sides.

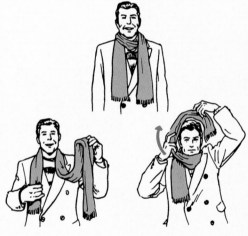

The Once Around

DRAPE THE scarf around your neck, leaving the right side short. Bring the left side over your shoulder and around your neck to the front.

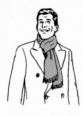

The Parisian Knot

FOLD THE scarf in half and drape it around your neck. Bring the loose ends through the loop and tighten.

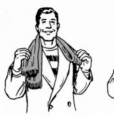
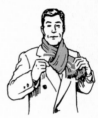

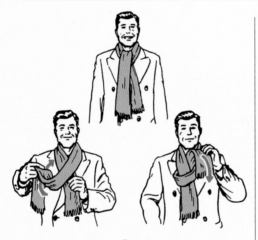

The Overhand

DRAPE THE scarf around your neck, leaving the right side short, and crossing the left side over it. Bring the left side up through the loop in the neck and back out the front.

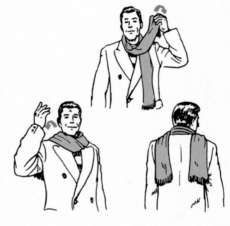

Reverse Drape

WITH THE scarf around your neck (equal lengths on both sides), take the right side and throw it over your left shoulder, and throw the left side over your right shoulder.

HOW A SUIT SHOULD FIT

While the number of jobs that require dressing up in a suit is declining, it's still common practice for many businesses—and a surefire way to look sharp. Whether you wear a suit five days a week or only dust it off for a special occasion, it should fit well. Not only do ill-fitting suits look bad, they're uncomfortable. From pinched arms to dragging pants, don't settle for suits that are too big or too small—get them tailored just right.

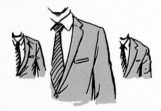

Shoulder

THE SHOULDER line should be smooth. Too tight and you'll see creases. Too loose and you'll have rumpled sections.

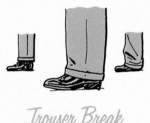

Trouser Break

PANTS SHOULD touch your shoe and crease slightly in the front only.

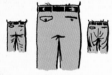

Seat

PANTS SHOULD drape over the seat. Look out for bunching or excessive fabric that causes a billowy look.

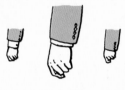

Sleeve Length

SLEEVES SHOULD allow half an inch of your shirt to show.

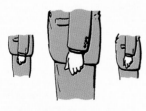

Jacket Length

YOUR JACKET should meet the middle of your palm when your arms are relaxed at your side.

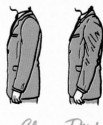

Sleeve Pitch

WITH ARMS relaxed, the sleeve fabric should be smooth, not twisted or bunched.

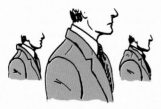

Jacket Collar

FIT THE collar to create a seamless transition between your neck and back. Avoid loose collars that pull away and tight collars that cause bunching.

Not only do ill-fitting suits look bad, they're uncomfortable.

MATCH A SHIRT AND TIE

Nothing throws off a put-together ensemble like a mismatched tie. Keep these guidelines in mind.

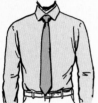
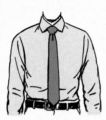

Analogous   *Contrasting*

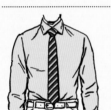
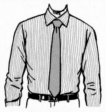

Patterned Tie with   *Solid Tie with*
Solid Shirt   *Patterned Shirt*

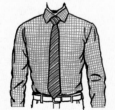

Striped Tie with
Checkered Shirt

1: BEGINNER—Match solid shirts with solid ties. Use contrasting shades of the same color, like a light-blue shirt with a dark-blue tie, or two contrasting colors, like a light-pink shirt with a navy-blue tie. When in doubt, set a solid color tie against a classic white shirt.

2: INTERMEDIATE—Match a patterned tie with a solid shirt or vice versa. The trick is to make sure there is a unifying or matching color between the shirt and tie.

3: ADVANCED—Match a patterned tie with a patterned shirt using these rules. One, the pattern styles must be different—like a striped tie with a checkered shirt. Two, the pattern sizes must be different. Don't match a tie with tiny polka dots with a shirt that has a tight plaid pattern. Three, ensure there is a unifying or matching color between the tie and shirt.

COORDINATE YOUR SHOES
WITH YOUR SUIT

Once you have your shirt and tie put together, you need to match your shoes to your suit. It's not that complicated—but remember, your belt should always be the same color as your shoes.

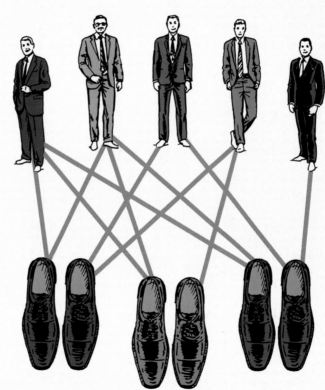

1: NAVY suit—
burgundy, brown, or
black shoes

2: LIGHT-GRAY suit—
burgundy, brown, or
black shoes

3: DARK-GRAY suit—
burgundy or black
shoes

4: BROWN suit—
burgundy or brown
shoes

5: BLACK suit—
black shoes

IRON A DRESS SHIRT

Growing up, dear old mom might have ironed your dress shirts whenever you needed it. But you shouldn't need to rely on someone else to help make a strong first impression. Wrinkles make you look sloppy and out of sorts. Well-pressed clothing announces that you have your stuff together—that you're a man of discipline who knows details matter. Ironing is easy: You can press a shirt in less than five minutes.

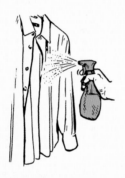

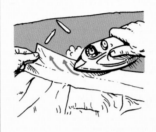

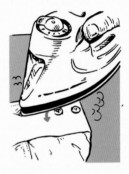

1: SLIGHTLY damp shirts are easier to iron than dry shirts. Remove the shirt from the dryer before it's fully dry or moisten it with a spritz of water. Look at the shirt's tag, and adjust the iron to the proper heat setting.

2: POP the collar and remove any collar tabs. Iron the underside of the collar first, slowly pressing the iron from one point to the other. Flip the shirt over and repeat on the other side.

3: IRON the cuffs. Unbutton one and lay it flat. Iron the inside first, then the outside, moving wrinkles from uneven fabric to the edges. Iron around the buttons, not over them.

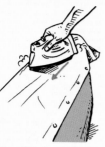

4: IRON the shirtfront. Start on the side with buttons and work the iron point around each one. Then move to the top of the shoulder and work your way down. Repeat on the other side.

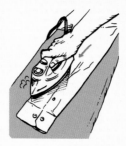

6: TIME for the sleeves. Take one sleeve by the seam and lay it flat on ironing board. If you can see the crease on the top of the sleeve from previous ironing, match it.

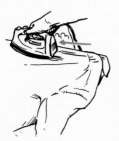

5: IRON the back. Start at the top with the yoke (back shoulder area) and slowly slide the iron down. If you have a center box pleat, spend a few seconds ironing around it.

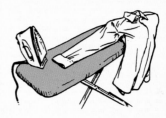

7: START ironing at the shoulder and work your way to the cuff. Turn the sleeve over and iron the opposite side, then repeat with the other sleeve.

ROLL YOUR SHIRT SLEEVES

Some sleeve-rolling techniques are more appropriate than others, depending on the garment and occasion.

WHEN SHOULD YOU ROLL YOUR SHIRT SLEEVES?

- When it's a practical necessity. Anytime they might get in the way, get dirty, or get caught in a moving part—roll 'em up.

- When it's hot outside. While the appropriateness of rolled sleeves varies by workplace, they're acceptable most times you have direct sunlight on your skin.

- When the situation calls for casual. Rolled sleeves dress down attire that would otherwise be too formal or dressy for the occasion; they send a signal that says "relaxed."

Suit or sport jackets usually aren't rolled (and when they are, they are more pushed up than rolled) unless there's an immediate and practical need. You can do it (if your jacket has working sleeve buttons), but be aware that it's a fashion-forward look.

The Basic Roll

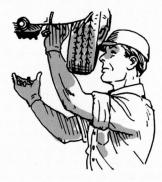

- **BEST** for: performing physical labor
- **BENEFITS:** simple and intuitive

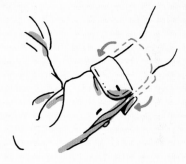

2: FLIP cuff back and inside out.

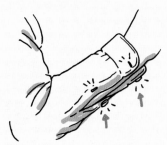

1: UNBUTTON cuff and any gauntlet buttons farther up sleeve.

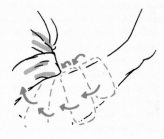

3: FOLD back, using the cuff to set the width, until band of rolled cloth is just below elbow—higher when engaging in physical labor.

The Casual Forearm Roll

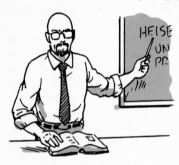

- **BEST** for: casual dress, thin arms, layers
- **BENEFITS:** involves the least folding, easiest to unroll without wrinkles

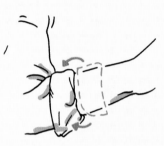

2: FOLD over once, hiding cuff behind a band of sleeve fabric.

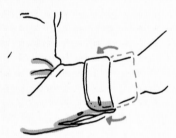

1: UNBUTTON cuff. Undo gauntlet buttons according to preference. Flip cuff back and inside out.

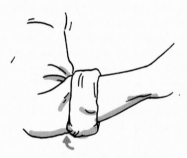

3: STOP there and tuck corners of cuff in neatly.

The Master/Italian Roll

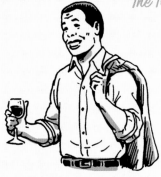

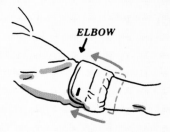

- **BEST** for: rolling sleeves with style, showing off cuffs with inner contrasting color
- **BENEFITS:** easy to adjust and unfold

2: PULL flipped cuff all the way to just below elbow without folding, turning sleeve inside out as it goes.

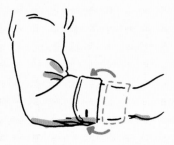

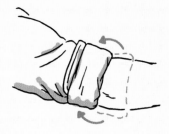

1: UNBUTTON cuff. Undo gauntlet buttons according to preference. Flip cuff back and inside out.

3: TAKE bottom of inside-out portion and fold it up until it traps bottom of cuff. Show as much of the inside-out cuff as you desire.

THE ART OF SHINING SHOES

Whether it's an upcoming wedding or graduation, or simply another day at the office, a pair of shiny shoes sets you apart as a man who cares about the details.

Not only does shining your shoes add panache to your appearance, it is a necessary part of properly caring for and maintaining a nice pair of leather shoes or boots. The polish helps moisturize and waterproof the leather, lengthening the lifespan of your shoes.

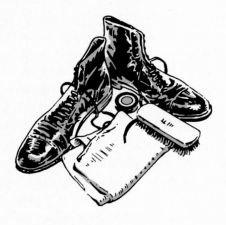

1: REMOVE any dirt/mud/salt with brush or damp rag. Wait until dry.

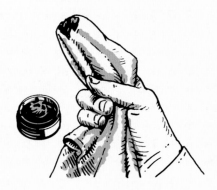

2: RUB a moist cloth in the polish to acquire a small amount on the cloth.

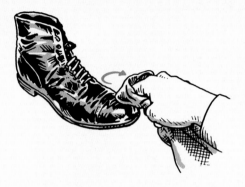

3: APPLY the polish in small circles, in small amounts.

Shining your shoes not only makes your shoes look good, but maintains them.

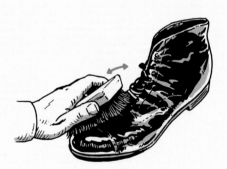

4: GRAB your shoe brush and brush the entire shoe vigorously.

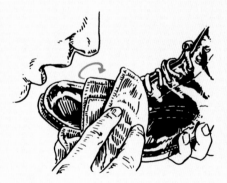

5: BREATHE "hot air" onto the shoe as if trying to fog a mirror on parts you want a really nice shine.

SHOE CARE 101

While regular shoe shining goes a long way in keeping your dress shoes in tip-top shape, it's not enough. To ensure that you get miles and miles out of your shoes, incorporate the following shoe care tactics into your routine.

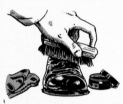

1: SHINE your shoes (page 72) after you buy them and before you wear them. Shine them regularly for as long as you own them.

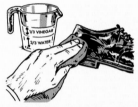

3: REMOVE a salt stain as quickly as possible by lightly applying a mixture of 2/3 water, 1/3 vinegar with a rag, wiping off with clean damp rag, and drying with a towel.

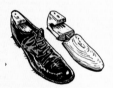

2: WHEN you remove your shoes, insert a cedar shoe tree to draw out inner moisture and reshape the leather.

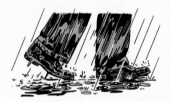

4: WATERPROOF your shoes with mink oil (may darken the color of the leather), a wax-based polish (light protection), or a specialty waterproofing compound (heavier protection).

5: CLEAN your shoes regularly to remove dirt, stains, and layers of built-up polish. Use a specialty leather cleaner, saddle soap, Murphy Oil Soap, or Ivory soap. Avoid products that contain detergents or acids.

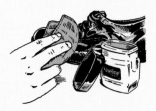

6: TO keep your shoes from drying out, every few months apply a specialty moisturizing conditioner or buff in a dab of petroleum jelly.

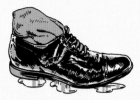

7: IF your shoes are wet, stuff them with newspaper or a small towel to draw out the moisture. Replace the paper/towels periodically as they get saturated. Never place your shoes near a heat source; this can dry out and crack the leather.

8: REMOVE scuff marks by rubbing the scuff with non-gel toothpaste. Rinse, wipe, and let dry.

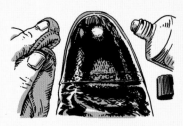

Note: The toothpaste trick does not work on every kind of shoe. Test the toothpaste on a small spot on the shoe to ensure compatibility with your particular leather.

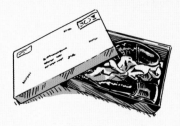

9: WHEN your shoes become really worn out, send them back to the manufacturer for refurbishing or resoling instead of buying a new pair.

ANATOMY OF A DOPP KIT

A traveling man needs only a few essentials to be happy. Nevertheless, you do need a place to stow these items. Enter the Dopp kit.

You can get a nylon travel bag for under $5 at any big box store; they'll get the job done. But if you want a Dopp kit with class, leather is the way to go. It will cost more, but last forever, age nicely, and become something you enjoy owning. It's something you might pass down to your son or grandson, along with the stories of the places you took it.

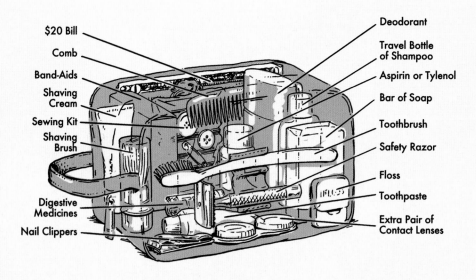

$20 Bill
Comb
Band-Aids
Shaving Cream
Sewing Kit
Shaving Brush
Digestive Medicines
Nail Clippers

Deodorant
Travel Bottle of Shampoo
Aspirin or Tylenol
Bar of Soap
Toothbrush
Safety Razor
Floss
Toothpaste
Extra Pair of Contact Lenses

THE GENTLEMAN'S ARSENAL

WHAT TO CARRY ON A DATE

Help ensure a date goes well by being well-prepared with both the intangible, like confidence and charisma, and the tangible, like an umbrella.

1: HANKIE—It's old school, but a clean linen handkerchief can mop up tears during a sad movie and wipe away spills at dinner.

2: CASH—Don't risk the chance that you'll encounter a business that only takes cash, leaving your date to pay for...your date.

3: MINTS—Take care of that garlic breath after dinner so you're ready for an up-close chitchat or a kiss.

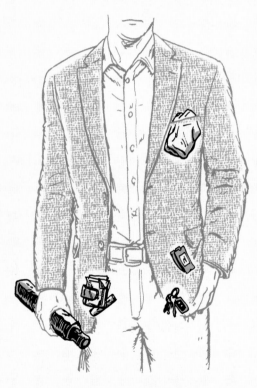

4: UMBRELLA—Check the weather before you go, and carry an umbrella in case the clouds open up.

5: SPORT coat—Dressed up or dressed down, a sport coat is the ultimate go-to clothing item for any date—and the perfect thing to offer your companion on a chilly walk.

SHAVE WITH A SAFETY RAZOR

Learning to shave is a rite of passage that has faded alongside the rise of expensive disposable cartridge razors and electric razors that require little skill to operate and deliver lackluster results. To get a close, smooth shave your grandpa would be proud of, go back to a double-edged safety razor—or skip right ahead to shaving with a straight razor (page 80).

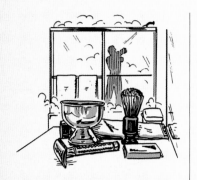

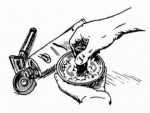

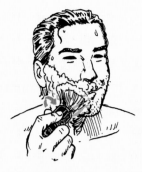

1: SOFTEN your facial hair by taking a shower or wetting your face with a hot towel.

2: PUT a dollop of shaving cream into a small cup and work it into a lather using your brush.

3: APPLY shaving cream to your face with the brush, completely covering your facial hair using swirling motions to create a smooth, even surface.

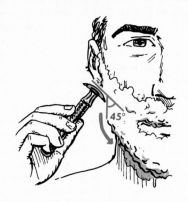

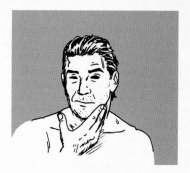

4: DRAG the safety razor with the grain of your hair, not against it, at a 45-degree angle, using only the pressure of the razor against your face.

5: GO for beard reduction rather than removal. You may not get everything on the first pass. Use multiple passes if needed to get the skin completely clear of hair.

If you must apply pressure to cut through your stubble, replace the blade —it's dull.

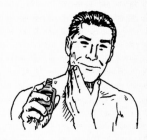

6: RINSE your face with cold water to close the pores. Apply your favorite aftershave to soothe your skin and reduce irritation.

SHAVE WITH A STRAIGHT RAZOR

Few things are manlier than taking a straight razor to the side of your face and deftly skimming off stubble. The straight razor is the samurai sword of shaving, but beyond its aesthetic and cool-factor benefits, it's the best way to get the closest shave with the least irritation. It's why high-end barbers still offer straight razor shaves to distinguished men needing a special shave before an important event or night out. Properly used, a straight razor will give you the best shave of your life.

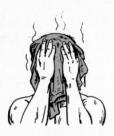 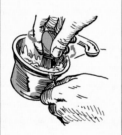 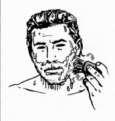 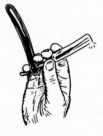

1: SOFTEN your facial hair by taking a shower or wetting your face with a hot towel.

2: PLACE a small amount of shaving cream into a small cup and work it into a lather using your brush.

3: APPLY shaving cream to your face with the brush, completely covering your facial hair using swirling motions to create a smooth, even surface.

4: HOLD the safety razor so that your thumb is alongside the blade, your pinky supporting the handle, and your three middle fingers supporting the back of the blade.

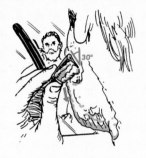

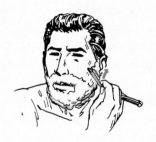

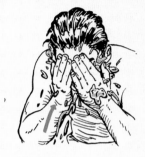

5: DRAW the blade with the grain of your facial hair at a 30-degree angle, using light pressure and even strokes.

6: REPEAT the process with more shaving cream, going across the grain of your hair on the second pass, and again with the grain of your hair on the third pass.

7: RINSE your face with cold water to close the pores. Apply your favorite aftershave to soothe your skin and reduce irritation.

Keep your razor sharp after each use by drying it and drawing it against a taut leather strop.

USE ALTERNATING strokes to drag the blade along the leather away from the blade's leading edge. Strop it before your next shave, as well.

TRIM AND STYLE YOUR MUSTACHE

If you decide to grow a cookie duster, you've got the responsibility of keeping it in tip-top shape so that it's presentable to the rest of the world.

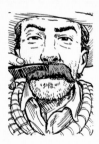 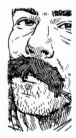 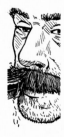 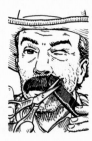

1: TRIM your mustache weekly. First, comb dry mustache with a fine-toothed mustache comb. When wet, hair can appear longer, leading you to cut off too much.

2: USING mustache scissors or an electric trimmer, trim first for shape, cutting along bottom of 'stache and then outer edges. Work from middle toward one side, then to other side and back to middle. Look straight ahead and maintain a neutral face to get a smooth, even line.

3: NOW trim for length. Comb through the 'stache and cut hair on the outside of the comb to desired length. Trim conservatively at first. If using an electric trimmer, move from longer to shorter guides. You can always trim off more, but you can't add it back after you've clipped it.

4: COMB through your mustache one last time, and clip any hairs you may have missed.

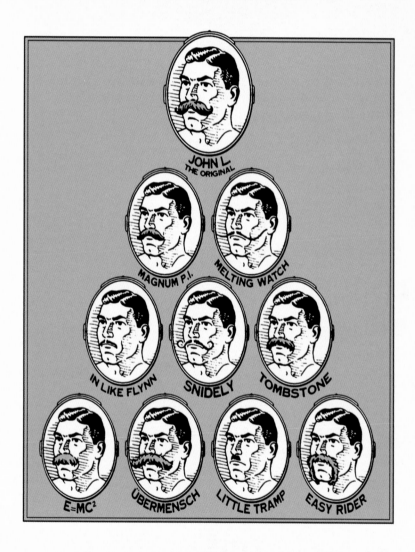

ROADMAP TO THE PERFECT FIRST DATE

First dates can be as terrifying as they are exciting. Figuring out what to wear, where to go, and what to do are challenging when you don't know someone very well. Remember, not all your first dates will go well. They're more about your connection with another person than they are about making the right dinner reservation. But with a little planning, you can alleviate the anxiety involved and create the atmosphere in which a perfect first date can happen. Above all, rely on these clichés that actually hold true—act with respect, be yourself, and have fun.

PREPARE

- Know where you're going and what you're going to do. Planning shows initiative and confidence.
- Clean your car and get some cash, just in case an activity pops up in which you need it.
- Dress appropriately, making sure your clothes are clean and ready well before your date.

PICKUP

- Arrive on time and be sure to notify your date in the unfortunate event that you're running late.
- Compliment her on the way she looks.
- Escort her from her door to your car and open the car door for her.

DRIVE

- Engage her in friendly conversation, asking her questions instead of talking about yourself.
- Don't crank up the tunes. If you want music, play something simple and pleasant, like old jazz.

DOOR

- Walk her to her door.
- Tell her you had a wonderful time and thank her for coming out.
- Offer a kiss or a hug if you feel it's appropriate, but don't make a move beyond that, even if she invites you in. You're a gentleman.

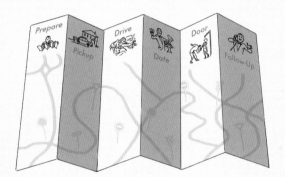

DATE

- Avoid the movies; you can't talk and learn more about each other.
- Do something active; a casual hike or a museum visit elicits conversation.
- Pay for everything.

FOLLOW-UP

- Call her the next day to thank her again for the date.
- At a later time, and if things went well, ask her if she'd like to go on a second date.

OPEN A DOOR FOR A WOMAN

Chivalry isn't dead. It's alive anytime a man goes out of his way to offer a helping hand, a kind gesture, or a sincere remark. Perhaps the easiest and most conventional way to display chivalry toward women is the act of opening a door. Some people in our modern, gender-egalitarian world think this tradition should be left in the dustbin of history. But if employed properly, chivalric rituals symbolize our differences as men and women while recognizing our equal worth. Rules and traditions give life texture and meaning. Sameness is boring. Difference creates attraction.

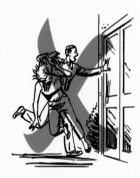

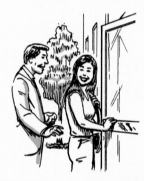

1: DON'T knock her over to get to the door first. Some men, eager to show off, will rush to the door to ensure they arrive before a woman does. Don't do that. The key to good manners is to make your efforts look effortless.

2: IF she doesn't want the door opened for her, respect that. Some women will tell you straight up that they don't like doors opened for them. Fair enough. Don't make a federal case of it.

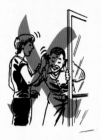

3: IF she starts opening the door for herself, just pull it open further. If your lady arrives at the door first and starts opening it on her own, all you need to do is to help pull the door open further. Don't brush her hand off the doorknob or door handle and don't offer any sanctimonious "I insist" or "allow me" entreaties. Don't make a big deal about it.

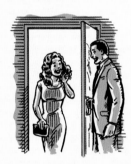

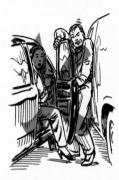

4: IF the door swings in, go through the door first and hold it for her. Doors that open inward are tricky. Go through these doors before your date does in order to hold the door open for her. If she arrives at the door first and begins pushing the door open, stand on the side of the door hinges and simply extend your arm over her head to take the door's weight from her as she passes through.

5: ONLY open car doors if there's nothing obstructing you. If there's not much room between your car and the car parked next to you, let her open her own door. Don't force a gesture it's just not possible to perform.

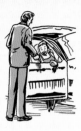

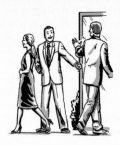

6: BEFORE shutting a car door, make sure all appendages, skirt bottoms, and purse straps are inside the vehicle. Don't ruin your date by slamming her foot in the door or tearing her dress.

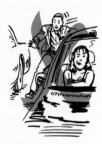

7: DON'T feel obligated to open the car door for her when exiting the vehicle. Most people get out of a car as soon as it parks. Opening a car door so your date can exit will probably require awkward maneuvering. You'll create a spectacle that may make your date feel like she's being chauffeured instead of courted.

8: OPEN doors regardless of gender. Holding doors open isn't something you need to do just for women. It's an act of common courtesy you can show to any person. A gentleman should always hold the door open for someone who is more physically burdened than he is. If you see an older person, a person with an obvious physical ailment, or a person holding a large package, hold the door.

And when someone opens a door for you, smile and say, "Thank you!"

LEARN TO DANCE

It takes two to tango. But whether you're looking to move to a lively salsa number, sway to the timeless sounds of a waltz or jazz standard, or start to swing—you need to start with the basics: the box step.

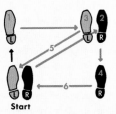

Start

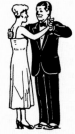

1: START with your feet together and your weight on your right foot.

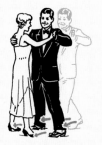

2: STEP forward with your left foot and then to the side on your right foot.

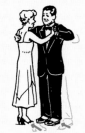

3: BRING your feet together and transfer your weight to your left foot.

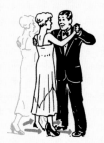

4: STEP back with your right foot and then to the side with your left foot.

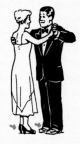

5: BRING your feet together and transfer your weight to your right foot to set up to begin again.

HELP A WOMAN WITH HER COAT

You've seen it in silver-screen classics. A dapper gentleman suavely and effortlessly helps his date put on her coat before they head out on the town. While your date is certainly capable of putting her own coat on, this is a simple way to show some consideration. But like opening a door for a woman, helping her put on her coat is easy to bungle—leaving both of you feeling awkward. Remember, the goal of courtesy is to make others feel comfortable, not awkward.

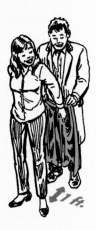
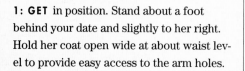
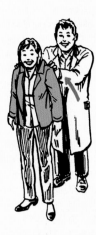

1: GET in position. Stand about a foot behind your date and slightly to her right. Hold her coat open wide at about waist level to provide easy access to the arm holes.

2: SLIDE the coat up. Once your date has her hands and wrists in the armholes, gently slide the coat up her arms and over her shoulders.

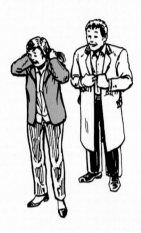

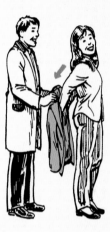

3: LET her do the finishing touches. Back away and let her button herself up and pull her hair out from beneath the coat collar.

4: REMOVING her coat. Removing her coat is simple. Just stand behind her and catch the coat as it slides off her shoulders. Hold it while she slides her arms out.

Remember, the goal of courtesy is to make others feel comfortable, not awkward.

TABLE MANNERS AND ETIQUETTE

Our society has become casual. But that doesn't mean manners can be thrown out the window when you're at the table with important guests. Learn the basics and practice at home, even if it means laying your napkin properly before scarfing down another slice of pizza on the couch.

GENERAL DINING ETIQUETTE

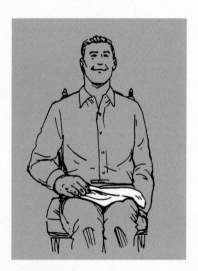

1: PLACE your napkin across your lap, bringing it out only to wipe your mouth as needed.

If you leave the table, place the napkin to the left of your plate until you return.

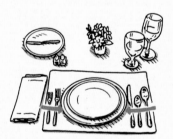

2: START by using the silverware at the outside of your place setting. As courses progress, use silverware closer to your plate.

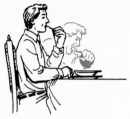

3: BRING food up to your mouth rather than leaning over, chew with your mouth closed, and do not talk while chewing.

Don't start eating until the majority of the table has begun.

WHEN ATTENDING A DINNER PARTY

Make an effort to try everything served by your host.

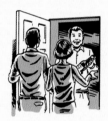

1: ALWAYS bring a gift, like flowers or a bottle of wine.

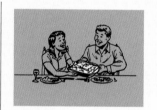

2: TAKE appropriately sized servings, making sure you leave enough for everyone, and always ask others to pass dishes that are out of your reach.

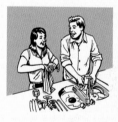

3: OFFER to help clean up and make sure to thank your host before leaving.

MASTER CLASSIC BAR TRICKS

These classic bar tricks, or "Tab Payers," inspired by *Esquire's* 1949 *Handbook for Hosts*, are alternately clever and goofy. Either way, you can use them to win a drink in a good-natured wager at the bar, or use them to break the ice at a party.

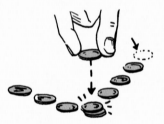

The Wager

THAT YOU can tell which way the match heads face in a closed match box.

The Payoff

BALANCE THE match box on a table knife; the side containing the match heads will be heavier.

The Wager

THAT IF you and a friend take turns picking up 1, 2, or 3 pennies from a pile, no matter how many pennies your companion picks up, you'll be able to make him draw last.

The Payoff

LAY DOWN a pile of exactly 17 pennies and ask your friend to pick first. Make sure the total number of pennies taken in each round is 4. If he takes 1, you take 3; if he takes 2, you take 2, if he takes 3, you take 1. You'll always win.

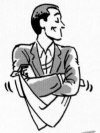

The Wager

THAT YOU can hold a napkin at the two ends and, without letting go, tie it into a knot.

The Payoff

FOLD YOUR arms before you grasp the ends of the napkin; when you unfold them the napkin will have a beautiful knot.

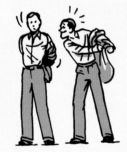

The Wager

THAT YOUR companion can't take off his coat by himself.

The Payoff

AS SOON as he begins, you start taking off your coat with him.

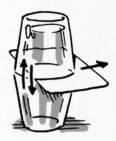

The Wager

FILL ONE shot glass with whiskey; fill a second shot glass with water. Offer to transfer all the whiskey into the water shot glass and all the water into the whiskey shot glass WITHOUT using a third vessel of any kind (including your mouth).

The Payoff

PLACE A business card over water glass, covering the rim completely. Turn it upside down, and place it on top of the whiskey glass. Pull the card out slightly to create a crack between the two glasses. The whiskey will slowly rise into the top glass and the water will sink into the bottom glass.

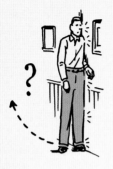

The Wager

THAT YOUR friend, standing with his left ankle, knee, hip, shoulder, and cheek pressed against the wall, can't lift his right leg off the floor.

The Payoff

HE CAN'T.

The Wager

THAT YOU can remove a dollar bill from under an inverted bottle without touching or upsetting the bottle.

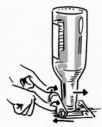

The Payoff

BEING CAREFUL not to touch the bottle with your hands, roll up the bill in such a way that the rolled portion gradually pushes the bottle off the bill and onto the table.

The Wager

THAT YOU can transfer water in a saucer to a glass without moving it.

The Payoff

HOLD A lighted match under the glass for a few moments; then place the inverted glass in the saucer and the water will mysteriously be drawn to it.

The Wager

THAT YOU can stay under water for any specified length of time.

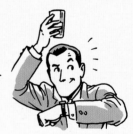

The Payoff

HOLD A glass of water over your head for the period agreed…then run, don't walk, to the closest exit.

Play the game for more than you can afford to lose . . . only then will you learn the game.

—Winston Churchill

GRILL A PERFECT STEAK

The smell of searing meat over an open flame brings us back to a primal state. Whether you prefer the fatty goodness of a ribeye, the lean and clean flavor of a flank, or a good old-fashioned T-bone, the keys to perfection are proper heat and timing.

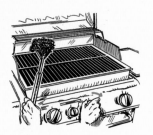

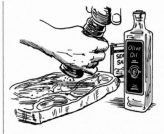

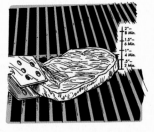

1: CLEAN and prepare your gas or charcoal grill for high, direct heat.

2: SEASON your steak with sea salt, fresh-ground pepper, and a little olive oil.

3: PLACE the steak directly on the grill grate. For every inch of steak thickness, cook each side for ~4 minutes.

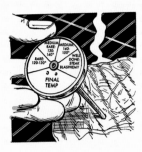

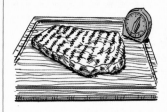

4: CHECK the temperature with a meat thermometer and pull the steak off 10 degrees before it hits your ideal final temp. It will continue cooking after you pull it off the grill.

5: ALLOW the steak to rest for at least half the time it was cooked.

6: CUT the steak against the grain for more tender slices. You can determine the direction of the grain by looking at which way the muscle fibers are running.

Determining a steak's grain may be easier before you grill it.

Chapter 3

The
TECHNICIAN

Craftsmanship means dwelling on a task for a long time and going deeply into it, because you want to get it right.

—Matthew B. Crawford

SINCE THE first humans start banging rocks together, man has cultivated an interest in tools. Tools make the inconceivable possible. Man the biological machine created artificial machines to do his work, keep him safe, communicate his ideas, and transport him across land and sea. The result is transformative new vistas explored, new foods eaten, new knowledge created, and new ways of living established.

Craftsmen, handymen, technicians—we depend on them because they make whole what is broken. Through skilled practice, a technician masters his tools in order to master the world around him. This mastery brings a deep sense of satisfaction and confidence that differs from the rewards of more ethereal "knowledge work." When you fix a leaky faucet or diagnose an engine problem, you see the immediate results of your action. The faucet stops leaking. The engine starts working.

In a culture that's fast outsourcing manual skills, a man needs to intentionally gain the proficiencies of a technician. These skills will help him become more self-reliant and useful to those around him, and connect his hands to the tangible world. Jump-start your apprenticeship in the following pages.

TOOLBOX ESSENTIALS

It's easy to tackle many jobs around the house when you have the right tools. Build your own tool kit and you'll have what you need to take on a variety of fix-it tasks. Avoid the urge to purchase all-in-one kits made of cheap metal. Instead, buy quality tools from reputable brands one at a time, and learn to use each one as you go. These are the essentials every toolbox should contain.

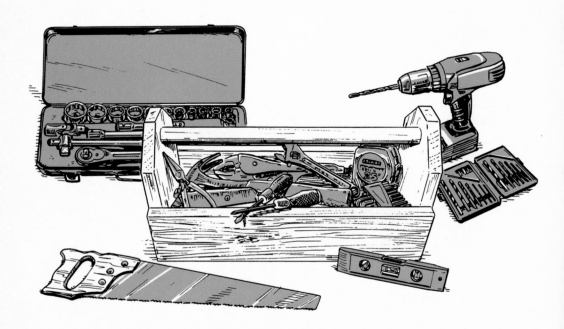

1: CLAW hammer—A 16-ounce hammer carries oomph without being unwieldy, and the claw on the back helps pry up old and bent nails.

2: SOCKET set—Nuts and bolts are no challenge for the ratcheting strength of a socket set. Sockets come in metric and imperial sizes. Get both.

3: NEEDLE-NOSE pliers— Get a pair with wire cutters for a dual-purpose tool.

4: CORDLESS drill and bits—Handy for drilling holes, driving screws, and a variety of other tasks, a cordless drill gives you power and flexibility.

5: CRESCENT wrench— Also known as a monkey wrench, this versatile nut and bolt turner is great for plumbing jobs.

6: TAPE measure—You'll be amazed at how often you need a tape measure in the garage and in the house. The 16-foot length covers most needs.

7: SCREWDRIVERS— Nearly all screws are of the Phillips-head or flathead variety. Pick out three sizes of each style with magnetic tips.

8: LEVEL— Hang perfectly straight pictures and avoid crooked lines whenever you're building. Longer levels are more accurate than short ones.

9: HANDSAW—A sharp saw will make basic cuts through wood, metal, plastic, and rubber.

10: ALLEN wrench set— From build-it-yourself furniture to bicycles, the six-sided grip of an Allen wrench (also known as a "hex key") is often in demand.

11: UTILITY knife—Ideal for opening hard plastic packaging and scoring wood, a sharp utility knife is a must-have tool you'll use a thousand different ways. Always store it with the blade retracted.

12: LOCKING pliers—Get a solid hold on just about anything with these powerful jaws.

HANDLE A HAMMER

Hammering may seem like the most basic tool technique known to man. But these tips can help avoid the frustration of bent nails and the pain of smashed fingers. Good technique will drive your targets in faster, so you can spend less time hammering and more time admiring your finished work.

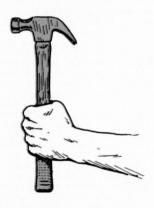

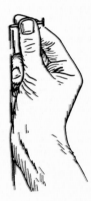

1: GRAB the hammer with a firm hand-shake grip. When starting a new nail, grip the hammer closer to the head for more control. As you drive the nail in, move your hand toward the bottom of the grip for increased power.

2: HOLD the nail between your thumb and forefinger, with the tip resting on the surface you're pounding it into. Grip the nail near the head to give you more control and prevent smashed fingers.

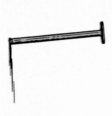

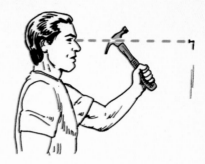

3: LIGHTLY tap the head of the nail with the hammer until the nail's tip digs in enough to hold it in place.

5: FOCUS your eyes on the nail head to avoid mishits and glancing blows.

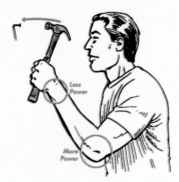

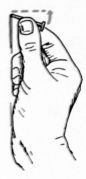

4: ADJUST your grip closer to the bottom of the hammer's handle and continue striking the nail. Use your wrist for light taps, transferring the power to your elbow as the nail is driven in.

6: PAUSE and re-align the nail if it starts to go in crooked. Fixing angled nails early improves your chances of getting the nail in straight.

USE A CRESCENT WRENCH

In its most simple form, a wrench is a tool that grips and turns things. And while most of us will only ever need to turn a crescent wrench or fiddle with a socket set, the complexity of professional wrenches and the nuts and bolts they turn is mind-boggling. The same basic principles for correct crescent wrench usage applies to almost all of them.

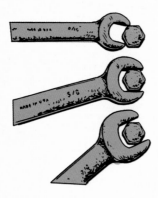

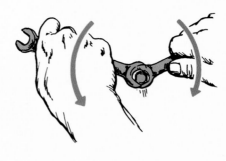

1: CHOOSE the correct size (or adjust it accordingly) to fit snugly on your nut or bolt. Wrench sizes and shapes can vary by mere millimeters, and using the wrong size can wreck the nut or bolt you're turning.

2: REMEMBER "righty tighty, lefty loosey." Turn clockwise to tighten and counter-clockwise to loosen.

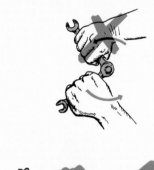

3: PULL, don't push, the wrench in the direction you want it to turn. Pushing may result in bruised knuckles if your nut or bolt breaks free suddenly.

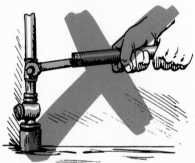

4: DON'T add leverage with a length of pipe. You may have seen your dad put a longer piece of pipe over his wrench to gain more leverage when tightening a fastener. You should avoid using "cheater bars" for several reasons. First, they can damage your wrench by bending the handle or jacking up the head. Second, because of the added torque you get with the extra leverage, you risk rounding your fastener if you don't have the right wrench head for the job. Finally, the cheater bar may slip off the wrench's handle while you're turning, causing harm to you or others. If you need more leverage, use a longer wrench.

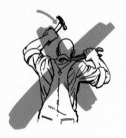

5: DON'T hit a wrench with a hammer. Unless you have a special "strike face" wrench that's designed for being hit with an object, you risk damaging your tools.

10 WAYS TO USE A POCKETKNIFE

From multi-toothed behemoths like the Swiss Army Knife to a simple penknife with a single blade that folds into a stylish handle, a knife expresses your personality while offering you reliable utility. Carry a knife and you're sure to use it for lots of things you never thought you would.

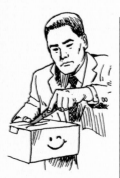

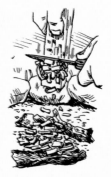

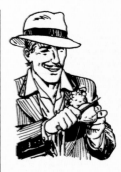

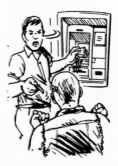

1: OPEN impossibly strong plastic packaging, boxes, and letters.

2: CREATE tinder from dry sticks for easy-to-start campfires.

3: CUT up food at a moment's notice.

4: DEFEND yourself against an attack.

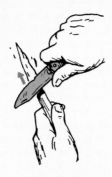

5: SHARPEN sticks into arrows or spears for survival.

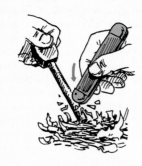

6: STRIKE a flint to create a spark to start a fire.

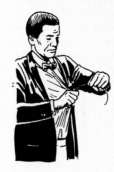

7: TRIM pesky loose strings and itchy tags on clothes.

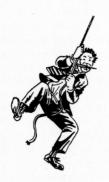

8: ACCESSORIZE by clenching the knife in your teeth while swinging from ropes, branches, and other Tarzan-approved apparatuses.

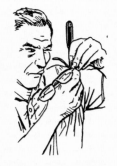

9: UNSCREW tiny flathead screws found in eyeglasses and small electronics.

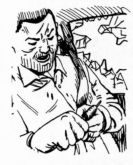

10: SLICE your seat belt off if it gets jammed after an accident.

SHARPEN A POCKETKNIFE

A knife's functionality is only as good as its maintenance. Although there are dozens of ways to sharpen knives, this basic technique goes a long way toward keeping your blade keen enough to do most jobs with ease. Sharp blades mean smoother cuts, which are safer because they require less force.

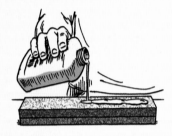

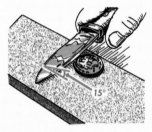

1: PREPARE a sharpening stone by lubricating the rough side with mineral oil. (Most stones have a smooth and a rough grit; start on the rough side.)

2: PLACE the blade against the stone so it makes a 15-degree angle.

Two quarters placed underneath the high edge of the blade will help set your knife at a 15-degree angle.

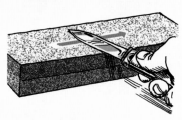

3: DRAG the blade across the stone, maintaining the angle throughout. Whether you drag the blade toward or away from you is a matter of personal preference.

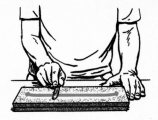

5: USE alternating passes to even out the edge on both sides of the blade. Drag one side of the blade and then the other, making approximately six more passes on each side.

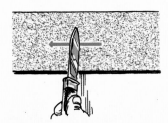

4: SWITCH to the other side of the blade after you make a dozen passes and repeat.

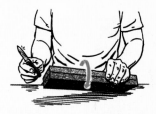

6: SWITCH to the smooth grit side of the stone and repeat steps 3 to 5.

Regular sharpening may only require that you use the smooth side of the stone.

A PRIMER ON AXES:
THEIR ANATOMY AND SAFE USE

If you were stranded in the wild or facing impending apocalypse, and could outfit yourself with one implement, you would be wise to choose the ax: part tool, part weapon.

Anatomy of an Ax

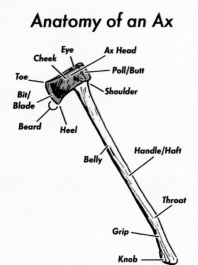

Eye
Cheek
Toe
Ax Head
Poll/Butt
Bit/ Blade
Shoulder
Beard
Heel
Belly
Handle/Haft
Throat
Grip
Knob

Double Bitted Ax

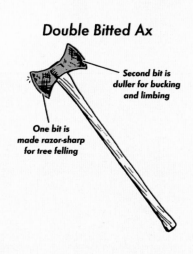

Second bit is duller for bucking and limbing

One bit is made razor-sharp for tree felling

Ax Safety

HOW TO STORE AN AX

Single Bit: Muzzle your ax!   *Double Bit*

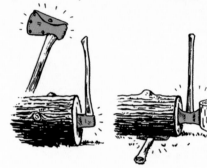

HOW TO CARRY AN AX

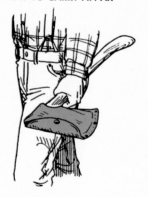

Felling a Tree

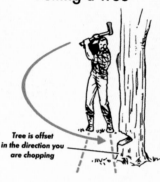

Tree is offset in the direction you are chopping

Bucking

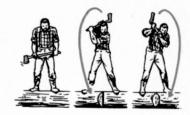

PICK A LOCK

Picking locks is the rare hobby that feels illegal even though it isn't. Beyond the utility this skill provides, it's a good lesson in safety. Pick your own locks and you'll realize the flaws in your home's security, which could lead you to consider other methods of theft-deterrence.

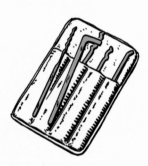

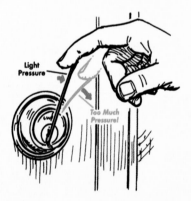

1: GET a basic lock-picking kit; one that's small enough to fit in your wallet is great. Choose one with a tension wrench and a basic rake.

2: INSERT the tension wrench into the keyhole and apply light pressure in the direction that the lock needs to turn. Use just enough pressure to hold the tension wrench in position.

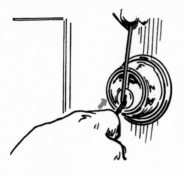

3: INSERT the rake in the keyhole at the top while maintaining pressure on the tension wrench.

Only pick locks on doors you have a legal right to open.

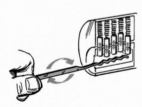

4: USE an elliptical motion to drag the rake along the upper interior of the lock.

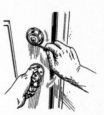

5: CONTINUE raking your pick and varying force on your tension wrench until the lock breaks free and the tension wrench turns the deadbolt.

TIE ESSENTIAL KNOTS

Beyond tying your shoes, it's altogether possible the only knots you know are the ones you make up on the spot. To the uninformed, complex knots seem like magic tricks. But you don't need to improvise the next time you lash something down. Practice this handy arsenal of knots instead.

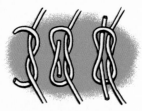 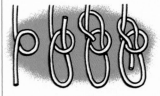 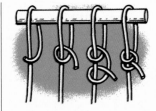

1: SQUARE knot—Also known as the reef knot, this is your best bet to connect two different ropes together for added length.

2: BOWLINE—One of the most important knots for sailors, this is perfect for forming a strong loop capable of holding heavy loads.

3: TWO half-hitches—This is ideal for tying anchor points or binding rope to objects, posts, and trees.

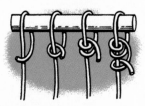

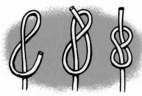

4: TAUT line hitch—Similar to the two half-hitches knot, this adds an adjustable hitch that allows you to lengthen or shorten your line under load. Perfect for attaching tent stakes to rainfly lines.

6: FIGURE eight knot—One of the simplest knots you can learn, this acts as a stopper for climbers and sailors who don't want ropes to slip out of retaining devices like pulleys.

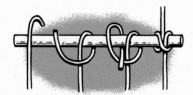

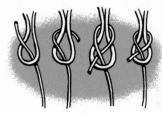

5: CLOVE hitch—Another binding knot, useful to create a solid anchor point and the best knot for tying logs together when making a raft.

7: SHEET bend—Use this instead of the square knot when you need to tie two ropes together, but the ropes are made of different materials or are different widths.

BREAK DOWN A DOOR

Kicking down a door is almost never the best way to open a locked door. Call a locksmith, pick the lock, or attempt to crawl in a window. But let's say it's an emergency. You're in a burning house and you need to escape through a locked door. You can't stand there fiddling with the lock! What to do? Be a man, dammit! Break down that door! You know you've always wanted to.

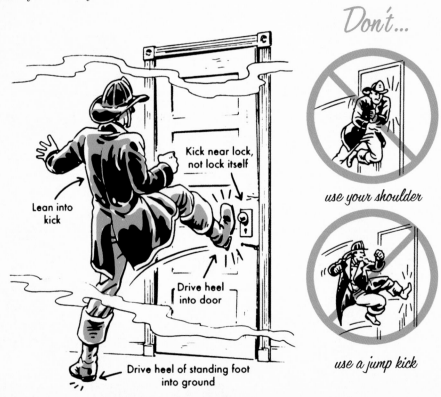

Don't...

Lean into kick

Kick near lock, not lock itself

Drive heel into door

Drive heel of standing foot into ground

use your shoulder

use a jump kick

THINGS EVERY MAN SHOULD KEEP IN THE CAR

Keeping these items in your vehicle can save you time and discomfort, and perhaps even your life, should emergency arise.

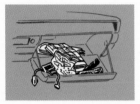 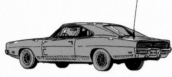 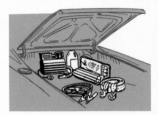

- Paper maps
- Snacks
- Seat belt cutter
- Flashlight

- Cell phone charger/extra charged battery

- Portable air compressor
- Windshield wiper fluid

- Roadside flares
- Jumper cables
- Tow strap

Additional Items for Winter and Emergencies

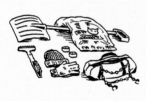

- Shovel
- Kitty litter
- Candles for heat
- Ice scraper
- Hat and gloves
- Tire chains

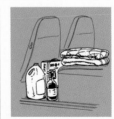

- Water
- First aid kit
- Warm blankets
- Small fire extinguisher

HOW A CAR ENGINE WORKS

If you use a car every day but have no clue how it works, today is the day that changes. Here is the heart of a car: the internal combustion engine.

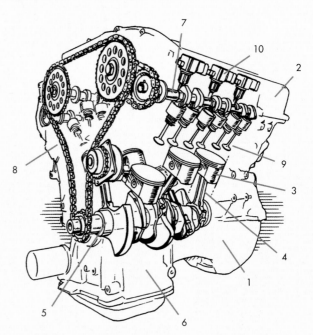

1: Engine block

2: Cylinder head

3: Piston

4: Connecting rod

5: Crankshaft

6: Crankcase

7: Camshaft

8: Timing chain

9: Valve

10: Spark plug

An internal combustion engine gets its name because fuel and air combust inside the engine to create energy to move pistons, which in turn move the car. This differs from an external combustion engine (like a steam engine), which is powered by energy created from burning fuel outside the engine.

ANATOMY OF A CAR ENGINE

Engine Block

THE ENGINE block is the foundation of an engine. Most are cast from aluminum alloy or iron. The engine block is also referred to as the cylinder block because of the cylinders that are cast into the structure. The cylinder is where the pistons slide up and down; the more cylinders an engine has the more powerful it is.

Combustion Chamber

THIS IS where the magic happens. Fuel, air, pressure, and electricity create a small explosion that moves the car's pistons up and down. The "walls" of the combustion chamber are made up of the cylinder, piston, and cylinder head.

Cylinder Head

THIS PIECE of metal sits over the engine's cylinders. A head gasket seals the joint between the cylinder head and cylinder block. Valves, spark plugs, and fuel injectors are also mounted to the cylinder head.

Piston

PISTONS MOVE up and down the cylinder and look like soup cans. When fuel ignites in the combustion chamber, the force pushes the piston down, which moves the crankshaft.

Crankshaft

THIS CONVERTS the motion of the pistons into rotational motion to move the car. At the front end, the crankshaft connects to belts that deliver power to other parts of the car via the camshaft; at the back, the crankshaft connects to the drive train, which transfers power to the wheels. At each end, oil seals called "O-rings" prevent oil from leaking.

THE CRANKSHAFT resides in the crankcase. The area at the bottom of a crankcase is the oil pan; that's where your engine's oil is stored. Inside, you'll find a pump that squirts oil onto the crankshaft, bearings, and cylinder walls to lubricate the piston stroke. The oil drips down into the pan to begin the process again.

Camshaft

THE CAMSHAFT is the brain of the engine. It works in conjunction with the crankshaft via a timing belt to open and close valves for optimal performance.

Timing System

THE CAMSHAFT and crankshaft coordinate their movements via a timing belt or chain, which holds them in the same relative position at all times.

Valves

INTAKE VALVES bring air and fuel into the combustion chamber. Outtake valves let out the exhaust from the combustion. Cars typically have one of each; most high-performing cars (like Jaguars or Maseratis) have four valves per cylinder. Multi-valve systems allow the car to "breathe" better, which improves engine performance.

Fuel Injectors

BEFORE THE 1980s, carburetors supplied fuel to the combustion chamber. Today, cars use direct fuel injection, which sprays fuel directly into the cylinder, or mixes fuel with air just before it enters the cylinder.

Spark Plug

ABOVE EACH cylinder is a spark plug. When it sparks, it ignites the compressed fuel and air, causing the mini-explosion that pushes the piston down.

THE FOUR-STROKE CYCLE

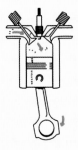 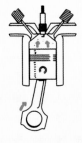 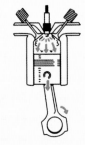 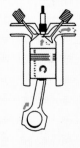

1: INTAKE Stroke. The piston lowers in the cylinder, sucking air into the cylinder through the intake valve while the fuel injector simultaneously sprays fuel in the cylinder.

2: COMPRESSION Stroke. The valves close, and crankshaft moves the piston up, compressing the air–fuel mixture.

3: COMBUSTION Stroke (Power Stroke). When the piston reaches the top, the spark plug sparks, igniting the air–fuel mixture. The resulting combustion forces the piston to the bottom of the cylinder again.

4: EXHAUST Stroke. When the piston reaches the bottom, the exhaust valve opens up. The piston comes back up, forcing the exhaust out of the cylinder.

DRIVE A STICK SHIFT

Driving with a stick shift is becoming a lost art. Today only 4% of new cars in the US are sold with manual transmissions. You never know when you'll need to know how to operate one. But the best reason to drive stick is that it's just plain fun.

GET FAMILIAR WITH YOUR COCKPIT

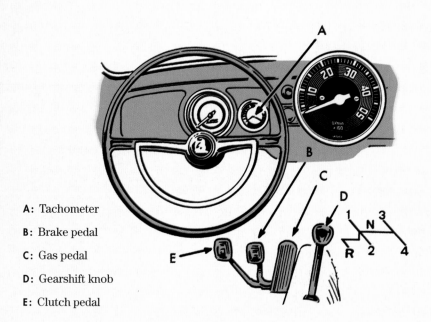

A: Tachometer

B: Brake pedal

C: Gas pedal

D: Gearshift knob

E: Clutch pedal

The pedals

CLUTCH, BRAKE, gas. The clutch pedal is on the far left; you press it when you shift gears. The brake is in the middle. The pedal on the right is the gas, and it works like the gas on an automatic transmission. You now have to use both feet when driving: your left foot to work the clutch and your right foot to press the brake and gas.

The gearshifter

MOST MODERN manual transmission vehicles come with six gears: first through fifth gears, and then reverse.

The tachometer

THE TACHOMETER shows you how many revolutions per minute your engine's crankshaft is going. Keep an eye on this; it will tell you generally when to shift gears.

GETTING THE CAR GOING

THE MOST intimidating part of driving a stick shift is getting the car into first gear. It takes a while to figure out how much you need to press down on the gas and how slowly you need to disengage the clutch for the gears to catch. Accept that you will stall the car. It's okay. It's your initiation into the Brotherhood of the Manual Transmission.

PRESS IN the clutch and brake pedal, and start the car. To start a manual transmission car, press the clutch while you turn the ignition switch. While you don't need to have your foot on the brake to start the car, it's a good habit to keep.

Starting the Car

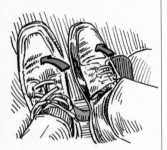
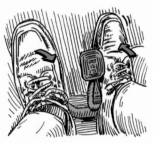
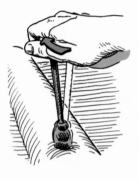

1: DEPRESS the clutch completely with your left foot and the brake with your right foot. Shift into first gear and start car.

2: SLOWLY lift left foot from clutch while pushing gently on gas with right foot.

3: NEVER shift gears without fully depressing the clutch pedal. Failing to do so will result in a horrific grinding sound and regular trips to the transmission shop.

When you drive with a stick shift you actually feel like you're part of the car, and you're attuned to its vibrations and noises. It makes driving a joy instead of a chore.

4: KEEP the clutch pedal and brake pushed down. Don't take your left foot off the clutch or you'll stall out. Keep the brake depressed as well.

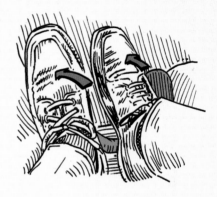

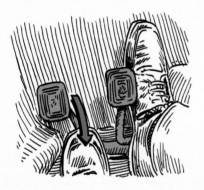

5: MOVE your right foot off the brake and onto the gas pedal. At the same time, start to release the clutch with your left foot. This is the tricky part. Slowly press the gas while you let up on the clutch. Don't stop pressing on the gas or you'll stall—keep light pressure on the pedal so the tachometer stays around 1,500–2,000 rpm. If all goes well, you should feel the gears "bite" or take hold of the spinning engine and you'll start slowly moving forward. When you're rolling, let up on the clutch completely.

6: COME to a stop. To stop, press down on the clutch with your left foot and the brake with your right foot at the same time.

7: THIS is the same process you'll use to back up, only you'll shift to reverse.

Shifting Gears

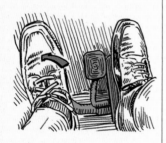

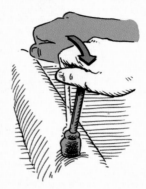

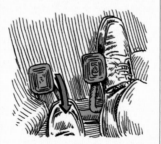

1: TAKE your right foot off the gas pedal, press in the clutch completely with your left foot, and shift into a lower or higher gear. This should be done in one synchronized motion.

2: REMOVE left foot from clutch while pressing on the gas pedal with right foot.

3: ONCE in gear, keep your foot off the clutch.

4: ONCE you get the car moving from a standstill into first gear, you've mastered 90% of stick shift driving. Upshifting into other gears is a breeze. Do it when the tachometer hits about 3,000 rpm. If you shift too soon, you'll feel the car shudder; downshift to keep it from stalling.

Practice in a parking lot when you're first starting out.

When you're ready to upshift:

1: TAKE your right foot off the gas pedal and press the clutch all the way down with left foot and move gearshifter fully to the next gear in one synchronized motion.

2: RELEASE clutch pedal while simultaneously pressing down on the gas pedal with right foot.

3: REMOVE your foot from the clutch pedal once you're in gear and continue to press the gas.

Use the same process to downshift as your car slows and the tachometer drops to around 1,000 rpm, but release your foot from the gas pedal.

Stopping

YOU CAN slow your car down by downshifting, but it takes a toll on your clutch and transmission. Instead, shift to neutral and use the brake, or press in the clutch and the brake at the same time.

Parking

THE EMERGENCY brake is your friend. Set it every time you park your car. For added safety, leave the car in first gear.

JUMP-START A CAR

Y̲ou never know when you'll need this knowledge to aid a friend, help a damsel in distress, or get yourself out of a jam. To avoid looking like a putz—or shocking yourself—when you jump a car, follow this guide.

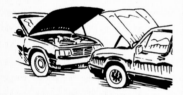

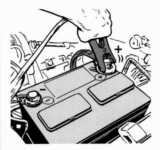

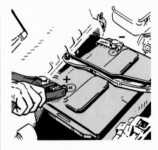

1: PULL jumper car next to car with dead battery. Make sure both cars are turned off and pop their hoods.

2: CONNECT one end of the red (positive) jumper cable to the positive terminal on the stalled battery.

3: CONNECT the other red (positive) cable clamp to the positive terminal of the good battery.

If you turn the ignition and hear the engine cranking, a dead battery isn't your problem and jump starting it won't do a darn thing. However, if you turn the key and the car does absolutely nothing, then there's a good chance you have a dead battery on your hands and jumping it may be your ticket to getting back on the road.

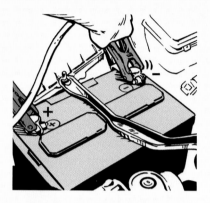

4: CONNECT one end of the black (negative) jumper cable to the negative terminal of the good battery.

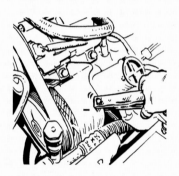

5: CONNECT the other black (negative) cable to a clean, unpainted metal surface under the disabled car's hood. Somewhere on the engine block is a good place. Do not connect the negative cable to the negative terminal of the dead battery.

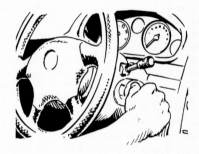

6: START the good car and run it for two to three minutes before starting the disabled car. Remove the cables in the reverse order of how you connected them. Keep the jumped car running for at least thirty minutes to recharge the battery.

CHANGE A FLAT TIRE

Maybe you have roadside assistance, maybe you don't. Either way, learn how to change a flat tire yourself. You never know when you, a loved one, or a stranger will need the help.

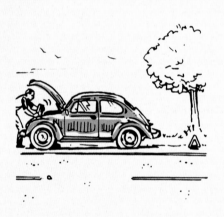
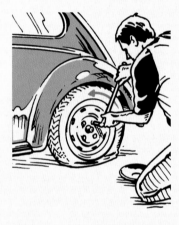

1: PARK car on flat surface, put on emergency brake and hazard lights, set up reflective warning triangle, put block on tire diagonally opposite flat tire, and remove spare tire from car (make sure it's inflated).

2: REMOVE hubcap so you can get to the lug nuts. Loosen nuts with lug wrench. Don't take any of them off yet—loosen just enough to "crack" them.

*Don't stick your hands or legs
under the car—it could fall and injure you.*

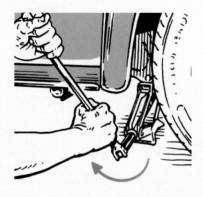

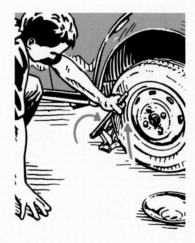

3: PLACE jack underneath car at a sturdy part of the frame. Check your owner's manual for correct placement. Turn crank at end of jack by hand until it contacts the frame.

4: ADD jack handle for leverage. Crank handle until wheel is high enough above the ground to remove the tire. Don't stick your hands or legs under the car—it could fall and injure you.

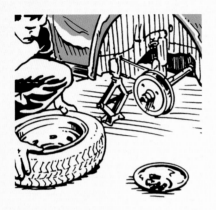

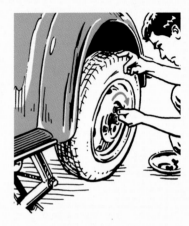

5: REMOVE lug nuts from wheel by turning them counterclockwise, and keep them in your hubcap so they don't roll away. Remove flat tire and lay flat. You don't want it to roll away, either.

6: LINE up spare tire with wheel studs and place on car. Once wheel is on, replace the lug nuts and tighten them by hand, and then with your lug wrench, until you meet firm resistance.

You can find specs on the proper torque for lug nuts in your car's owner's manual.

*Don't forget to put your tools away properly
for the next time!*

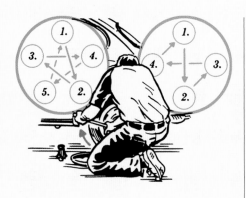

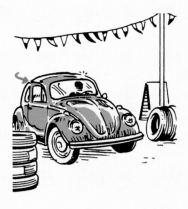

7: LOWER jack until wheel is firmly on the ground. Finish tightening your lug nuts. To get the lug nuts on as tightly as possible, unleash the power of the star pattern.

8: SPARE tires aren't supposed to be driven on for long distances or at high speeds, so you need to drive slowly and get your flat tire fixed and replaced as soon as possible.

CONTROL CAR SKIDS

Annually, over 100,000 injuries occur from car accidents on snowy or icy pavement. It's vital to have the skills necessary for driving safely in inclement conditions. Here are the five most common skids and how to recover from them.

1. WHEELSPIN

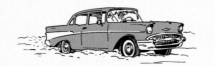

Take foot off gas.

WHEELSPIN OCCURS when you accelerate too quickly for the available traction. The tires will start to spin at a faster rate than the vehicle is actually traveling. The cure is simple: just back off the throttle until the tires regain traction, and ramp up more slowly next time.

2. WHEEL LOCKUP

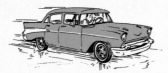

Take foot off brake.

WHEEL LOCKUP occurs when you brake too aggressively for the surface you're on: the tires will stop turning while the vehicle continues to move. The solution is to release the brakes until the tires start to turn again. You may need to release the brakes completely, and brake again more softly.

You can often brake fairly hard on a slippery road, as long as you do it smoothly. If you suddenly go from 0% to 50% brake on the snow, for example, they may lock up. But if you build up brake pressure progressively, you might brake well beyond 50% on the same surface.

ANTI-LOCK BRAKE Systems (ABS) will not allow your wheels to lock up; they'll pulsate brake pressure at all four wheels so that the tires keep turning. On a loose surface, your car may not decelerate very well, and you'll need to leave extra braking and following distances to compensate.

3. UNDERSTEER

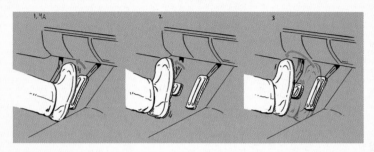

Take foot off gas and gently apply brakes. Slightly steer where you want to go.
You have the most grip with slight steering inputs.

AN UNDERSTEER skid occurs when the front tires lose grip, and the car is unable to turn a corner. It's also referred to as "plowing" or "pushing," and it occurs when you enter a corner with too much speed for the conditions. If you're doing 70 mph in a 30 mph corner, unfortunately it's all over… hope for something soft to hit. If you're only slightly too hot coming into a corner, let off of the gas and apply the brakes gently, while looking where you want the car to go at all times.

SPINNING THE front tires can also cause understeer. In a front-wheel drive car, don't spin the tires if you want to have any chance of turning. Locking the front tires will also cause understeer; if you're braking aggressively in any vehicle and trying to turn, you'll need to release the brakes somewhat in order to steer the car.

RESIST THE temptation to give the car more actual steering when you enter an understeer skid. It's the natural thing to do—"The car won't turn, so I'll turn more!"—but the problem needs to be fixed with the pedals and not with your hands. You have the best grip with slight steering inputs—if your front tires are turned at high angles there's very little chance they'll do what you want.

4. OVERSTEER

- *Rear-Drive Biased Cars—Take foot off gas.*

- *Front-Drive Biased Cars—Take foot off of brakes and gently apply gas.*

- *Slightly steer where you want to go.*
You have the most grip with slight steering inputs.

AN OVERSTEER skid occurs when the rear tires lose grip, and the rear of the vehicle starts to slide sideways. This often occurs because of wheelspin in rear-wheel drive (and some all-wheel drive) vehicles, and the solution in that case is to back off the throttle, look where you want to go, and slightly steer in that direction.

OVERSTEER ALSO occurs fairly often when you're going too fast for the conditions, and apply brakes while turning a corner. This will shift much of the vehicle's weight onto the front tires and off of the rear. The rear will start to come around simply because there is no weight on those tires, especially in pickup trucks, front-wheel-drive cars, or other vehicles that are naturally light in the back. This happens going downhill around corners for the same reason. Again, the solution is to look down the road where you want to go, release the brakes, and even accelerate a little to put some weight back onto the rear tires to stop them from sliding.

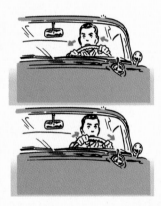

5. COUNTERSKID

- *Rear-Drive Biased Cars—Take foot off gas.*

- *Front-Drive Biased Cars—Take foot off of brakes and gently apply gas.*

- *Slightly steer where you want to go.*
You have the most grip with slight steering inputs.

- *As the vehicle straightens out,*
straighten the wheel so that the tires are always pointed down the road.

KNOWN AS "fishtailing" or "tankslapping," counterskids occur when you have met with oversteer and failed to correct appropriately. The rear end of the vehicle skids back and forth, often building momentum with each swing. If you don't fix the first or second skid, you'll often generate enough energy to make the third skid violent and difficult to recover from. Take your feet off

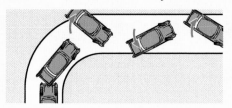

both pedals and focus on catching up on the steering. Braking or accelerating will just compound your problems.

LOOK DOWN the road and only use enough corrective steering to point the front tires where you want to go. As the vehicle straightens out, straighten the wheel so that the tires are always pointed down the road. Counterskids most often happen when drivers correct late, overcorrect, and then repeat this mistake until they're off the road. Your vision is the key. Regain control of the steering, don't let the car bounce back and forth, and you'll be fine.

Chapter 4

The WARRIOR

Unless we keep the barbarian virtues,
gaining the civilized ones will be of little avail.

—Theodore Roosevelt

MEN ARE hardwired to fight and defend. The ancient world was a rough and dangerous place. Men who were able to protect themselves lived to pass on their genes to the next generation. The blood of this lineage of warriors runs through the veins of men today. But thanks to the advances of modernity, most of us no longer need to be full-time fighters. We have the luxury of outsourcing our protection to a small class of professional warriors that serve in military and police forces.

YET THE ANCIENT CALL OF THE WARRIOR STILL BECKONS.

Every man has probably asked himself, "Would I be able to protect myself or my loved ones if I had to?" We live in a relatively safe and peaceful time, but attacks and assaults still occur. And when danger strikes, it often strikes suddenly, with no time to call the police. This chapter helps you stand a fighting chance.

DO A LOW BAR SQUAT

The squat is one of the most basic human movements, and calls upon some of the largest muscles in the body. If you want to be as strong as possible, you want to work as many of these large muscles as possible. Enter the low bar squat.

When most folks squat at the gym, they likely use the high bar squat, in which the bar is placed high on the trapezius and an upright torso is maintained throughout the lift. There's a place for the high bar squat in strength training routines, but if you want to work more muscles in the posterior chain as well as lift more weight, the low bar squat can't be beat.

SET-UP

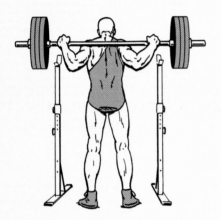

1. **BAR** is placed just beneath the spine of the scapula
2. **ELBOWS** up
3. **CHEST** up
4. **THUMBS** on top of the bar
5. **HANDS** as close together as flexibility allows
6. **FEET** about shoulder-width apart
7. **TOES** pointed out about 30–35 degrees

DESCENT

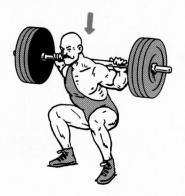

1: LEAN over a bit—point your nipples to the floor

2: EYES and head look down

3: SHOVE knees out

4: TAKE big breath before descending and hold during entire lift

5: GO down to parallel—crease of the hips will be about an inch below the top of the knee

6: WEIGHT should be in the middle of the foot throughout entire lift

ASCENT

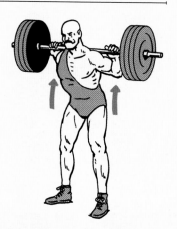

1: DRIVE up with hips

2: KEEP head and eyes looking down

3: SHOULDER and hips should rise up at the same time to maintain bent over back angle

4: EXHALE when the lift is done

DEADLIFT

The deadlift is a deceptively simple exercise—just lift a weighted barbell off the ground until you're standing upright. But don't let its simplicity fool you. While it's primarily a back exercise, the deadlift calls upon other muscles like your core, shoulders and traps, and forearms. It's a full-body exercise.

Besides being highly functional, the deadlift is just plain fun to do. Nothing makes you feel manlier than pulling hundreds of pounds off the floor.

START

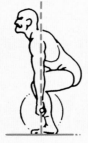 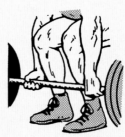

1: SHOULDERS in front of bar

2: ARMS vertical to floor outside of knees

3: BEND knees until shins hit bar

4: STAND with bar above the center of your feet

5: RAISE hips until you feel hamstring tension

6: FEET slightly more than hip-width apart, pointed straight ahead or slightly outward

7: HANDS about shoulder-width apart with overhand grip OR optional overhand/underhand grip

LIFT

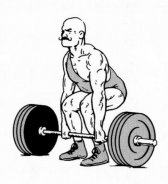

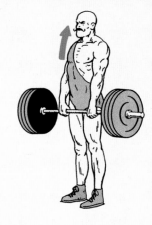

1: **HEAD** in line with spine, chin up, looking straight ahead

2: **LIFT** your chest but don't squeeze your shoulder blades

3: **BACK** erect with slight arch. DO NOT ROUND OR FLATTEN BACK

4: **KEEP** bar close to body—roll it over your knees and thigh until hips and knees are locked

5: **DO** not lean backward or bend forward

6: **DRIVE** heels into floor and push up with legs

LOWER

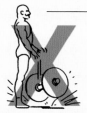

1: **PUSH** hips back first, and then bend your knees once bar reaches knee level, keeping bar close to body. Don't drop it!

USE A KETTLEBELL

Kettlebells look like a cannonball with a handle, and they've been used by Russian strong-men for over two centuries to "become strong like bull." They're one of the most versa-tile pieces of training equipment known to man and will give you the workout of your life.

SUMO DEADLIFT

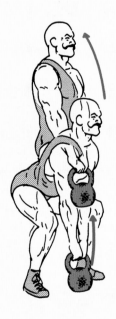

1: STAND over your kettlebell with your feet slightly wider than shoulder-width apart. Have your feet turned out just a bit. Sit back as if you were going to sit in a chair or crap in the woods. Keep your heels firmly planted on the ground. No tippy toes. Pick up the kettlebell with both hands, keeping your arms straight. Your shoulders shouldn't be ahead of your knees. Keeping your back and arms straight, lift the kettlebell off the ground with your legs until you're standing straight up. Do not bend your arms as you stand, and do not lift with your back. When you're in the standing position, your body should form a straight line. Lower the kettlebell back to the ground. Repeat ten to twenty times.

TWO-ARM SWING

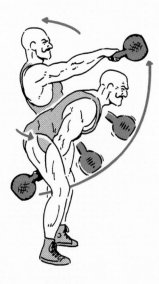

1: STAND above your kettlebell with your feet shoulder-width apart and the bell between your heels. Lower your hips as if you were going to sit down in a chair and grab the kettlebell with both hands. Arms should be straight; shoulders behind knees;

back straight. Make sure your weight is on your heels—not your toes. Basically you're doing the starting position of a sumo squat.

2: POP your hips forward to get the kettlebell to swing out in front of you a bit. You basically want to "hump" the air in front of you.

3: LET the kettlebell swing back behind your butt like you were snapping a football to a quarterback. When the bell is by your butt, explosively drive your hips forward (hump that air!) and swing the kettlebell up to chest level. Keep your arms straight and relaxed during the swing up. When the kettlebell reaches chest level, let your arms swing back down so that the kettlebell goes back to your butt. Drive your hips forward for another swing. Repeat. Make sure you keep your head up and back straight during your swings.

4: YOU can swing for time or for reps.

CLEAN AND PRESS

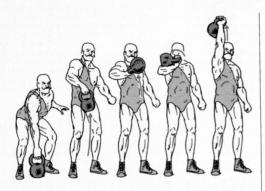

1: STRADDLE the kettlebell with your feet a little wider than shoulder-width apart and slightly pointed out. Squat down and grasp the kettlebell's handle with one hand in an overhand grip. Position your shoulder over the kettlebell while keeping your back straight and looking forward.

2: THE following is done in one motion. Inhale and pull kettlebell up off the floor by bringing your hips forward. Once kettlebell is off the ground, vigorously pull it up with your shoulder, allowing your elbow to bend out to your side. Imagine you're pulling the starter cord on a lawnmower. Keep the kettlebell as close to your body as you can.

3: WHEN the kettlebell reaches about chest level, rotate your elbow under the bell. Catch the kettlebell on the outside of your arm; wrist is straight and knees are slightly bent. The bell will end up between your forearm and biceps. This is called the "rack position." Exhale. Some folks (like me) like to do a full-on front squat instead of slightly bending their knees. I prefer this method because it gives my quads a nice workout.

4: INHALE and explosively press the kettlebell off your arm and straight up to lock-out over your head. Exhale when you reach lock-out.

5: LOWER the kettlebell back to the rack position. Slowly lower the kettlebell to the ground between your legs while squatting down, keeping your back straight, and your head looking forward. Repeat.

TURKISH GET-UP

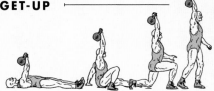

THE TURKISH Get-up looks easy, but—holy smokes—it's a killer exercise. Start off with a lighter kettlebell when you first start doing it. As you proceed, keep the arm that's holding the kettlebell straight and your eyes on the weight during the entire lift. Take it slow and be deliberate with your movements.

1: LIE down on your back. Hold the kettlebell in your right hand and fully extend your right arm above you so that you're holding the kettlebell above your chest. Your shoulder should be tight in the socket. To achieve this, think about "packing" your shoulder blade down and back. Your lat should be touching the ground.

2: BEND your right leg at your knee so that your right heel is near your butt. Keep your left leg straight. Place your left arm out to the side, palm facedown on the ground. Keep your right arm fully extended above your head and your eyes on the kettlebell.

3: BEGIN to lift your right shoulder off the ground and come up and rest on your left elbow. Keep the kettlebell above you, held by your fully extended right arm. Keep your chest up and out.

4: TRANSITION from your left elbow to your left hand. Focus on keeping that right arm fully extended. Continue that good posture by keeping the chest up and out.

5: DRIVE your hips upward and squeeze those glutes. You should now be in a bridge position with just your left hand and both feet on the ground. Your right arm is still fully extended and your eyes are on the weight.

6: SWEEP your extended left leg back behind your body so that your left knee is on the ground. You should be in a lunging position. Torso should be erect. Keep that right arm extended.

7: NOW stand up. It's the same movement as if you were rising from a lunge. Again, keep your right arm straight. Congratulations! You just completed one repetition of a Turkish Get-up. Follow these steps in reverse to return to the starting position on your back. Go for five to ten reps. Switch sides and perform the lift on your left side.

DO THE PERFECT PUSH-UP

It's hard to beat the classic burn of an old school push-up. But while most people have been doing push-ups since their first P.E. class, mastering the subtleties can help you get the most out of this exercise. Pay attention to the details and push your way to a stronger body.

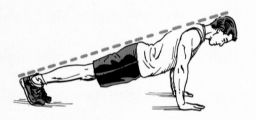

- Position hands directly under shoulders
- Keep your feet together
- Align your legs, spine, and neck
- Clench your glutes

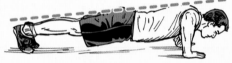

- Lower until your chest grazes the floor
- Keep your core engaged as you start to push back up

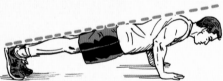

- Inhale as you lower to the ground
- Keep your biceps close to your body
- Maintain a straight line along legs, spine, and neck

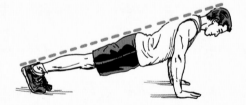

- Exhale when you push back up
- Don't lock elbows at top; maintain some muscle tension

DO THE PERFECT PULL-UP

Pull-ups are one of the best ways to make serious strength gains without a mess of equipment. Done wrong, they can also wreak havoc on your back, joints, and tendons throughout your arms. Get a grip on the proper technique with these steps.

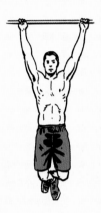
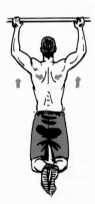

- Position your hands facing away from you, and slightly more than shoulder-width apart

- Cross your feet to help stabilize your legs

- Pull your shoulder blades together to start movement using your back muscles, rather than your arms

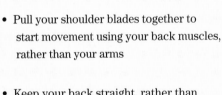

- Keep your back straight, rather than arching it
- Flex your abs and glutes to prevent your legs from swinging

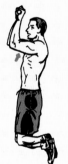
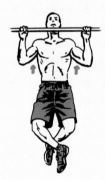

- Pull with your entire upper body, rather than relying on your arms alone
- Clear the bar completely with your chin before lowering slowly into your hanging position

PRISONER WORKOUTS

Prisoners all over the world have created effective strength-building routines they can perform in their cells or with limited equipment in the jail yard. We can all take a lesson not to let our circumstances excuse our fitness goals. Bodyweight exercises, ranging from push-ups, pull-ups, and dips, to squats, leg raises, and burpees, are an excellent way to build strength and endurance wherever you are. Try these prison workout techniques on for size. (Warning: Due to the high reps of these workouts, precaution should be taken lest you end up in the hospital with rhabdomyolysis. Start slow and don't push yourself too hard at the beginning.)

DECK OF PAIN

1: TAKE a standard deck of fifty-two cards. Assign a bodyweight exercise to each of the four suits. For instance: clubs = push-ups, spades = pull-ups, diamonds = squats, and hearts = hanging leg raises.

2: START drawing cards from the top. The suit tells you what exercise you're doing; the number tells you the reps. Face cards count as ten; aces, eleven. Keep drawing and exercising until all the cards have been drawn.

3: FINISH it off with ten burpees for good measure. Be careful with this routine. The high repetitions it involves can induce rhabdomyolysis—when your muscles work so hard they basically turn into dust and get into your bloodstream. It can be lethal.

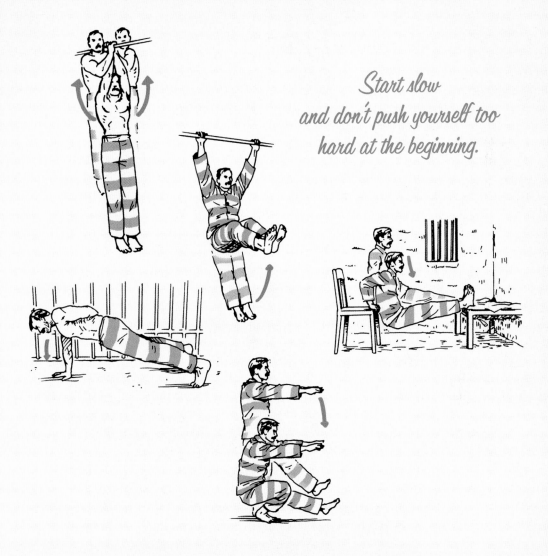

Start slow
and don't push yourself too
hard at the beginning.

JUAREZ VALLEY METHOD

1: ACCORDING to the book Jailhouse Strong, the convicts inside Mexico's Juarez Valley Prison—one of the world's most dangerous—use this rep scheme for their bodyweight workouts.

2: PICK an exercise. You're only going to do one during this circuit. Let's say for this example, you're going to do push-ups. The circuit consists of 20 sets. The rep scheme looks like this:

- Set 1: 20 reps
- Set 2: 1 rep
- Set 3: 19 reps
- Set 4: 2 reps
- Set 5: 18 reps
- Set 6: 3 reps
- Set 7: 17 reps
- Set 8: 4 reps
- Set 9: 16 reps
- Set 10: 5 reps
- Set 11: 15 reps
- Set 12: 6 reps
- Set 13: 14 reps
- Set 14: 7 reps
- Set 15: 13 reps
- Set 16: 8 reps
- Set 17: 12 reps
- Set 18: 9 reps
- Set 19: 11 reps
- Set 20: 10 reps

3: ON the odd sets, you start with 20 reps and count down, and on the even sets, you start from 1 rep and count up. Between each set, walk 5–10 steps for a rest and then get back into it. The goal is to complete this circuit as fast as you can. By the end, you've completed 210 reps.

All you need is a tolerance for pain and a drive to improve.

*Everyone has a plan until they get
punched in the mouth.*

—Mike Tyson

MIKE TYSON SQUAT WORKOUT

TYSON DID this routine while in prison. It doesn't sound hard but it's a real killer.

LINE UP ten cards facedown in a straight line on the ground with four inches between each card. Begin by standing over the first card, squat down, and pick up the first card. Holding the first card, take a step to the second card. Squat down and place the card you just picked up on top of the second card. At this point, you have no cards in your hand, and two cards will be one on top of the other on the ground below you.

THEN SQUAT once and pick up the top card. Squat again and pick up the card that was on the bottom. Take a step forward to the third card, squat down, and place one of the two cards in your hand on top of the card on the ground. Now squat down and place the other card on top of the cards on the ground.

SQUAT ONE time each to pick up the three cards one by one. Take a step forward to the fourth card, and repeat this process until you've made it through all ten cards.

THROW A STRAIGHT PUNCH

The straight punch, or cross, is a devastating power punch that leaves you in a good position to follow up with other punches. But for it to be effective, you've got to do it correctly. Here's how.

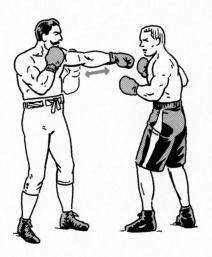

1: OPEN opponent up with some high jabs and a few fakes.

2: END sequence with jab from your non-dominant hand so your dominant hand is ready to throw the straight punch.

3: WHEN your opponent drops his guard, you're ready to throw your dynamite punch.

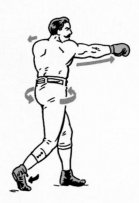

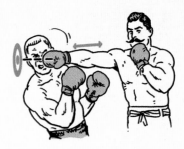

1: BRING shoulder and jab hand back while simultaneously throwing the straight punch with your dominant hand.

2: DON'T broadcast the punch; keep elbow in.

3: INCREASE your punch's power by pushing off back foot and twisting hips much like you would swing a baseball bat.

4: DRIVE toes into ground like you're squishing a bug.

5: RIGHT knee points at left knee.

1: FOR maximum power, don't aim at your opponent's face, but behind it.

2: PUNCH straight out and straight back.

3: KEEP jab hand up to protect against any counters.

THROW AN UPPERCUT

As one of the most powerful punches in a boxer's arsenal, the uppercut is a tool not to be taken lightly, or thrown without consideration. Usually reserved for the end of a combination of jabs and crosses, uppercut punches are best used when you're close to your opponent and have an opening at their chin or solar plexus. As with any punch, a good uppercut starts with a solid stance and finishes with a smooth transfer of weight and power.

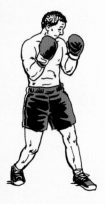 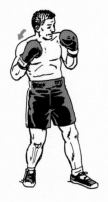 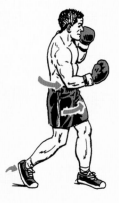 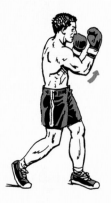

1: START with a strong stance, with your non-dominant foot forward and weight on your toes.

2: ADJUST your shoulders so that they angle down toward your punching arm.

3: LEAD the punch with your hips, moving them forward and up as your back foot lifts up.

4: ROTATE through the shoulders, keeping your elbow behind your wrist as you come across and up through the punch.

THE TACTICAL ORDER OF GETTING DRESSED

Military and emergency personnel are taught the most efficient order in which to dress because they must be out the door in seconds. To help you do likewise when the need arises, we present two tactical methods used by soldiers and first responders.

SPEEDY

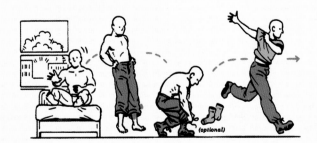

1: PANTS

2: BOOTS

Socks (optional)

3: SHIRT

(optional)

SPEEDIER

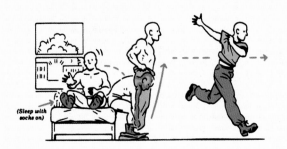

1: **BOOTS** inside Pant Legs

2: SHIRT

Sleep with socks on.

(Sleep with socks on)

FIRE A GUN

Handling a firearm is an awesome responsibility that must be taken seriously; terrible damage can be done. There's no room for carelessness. In addition to reading this guide, seek safety training from a real professional before pulling the trigger.

THE FOUR CARDINAL SAFETY RULES OF FIRING ANY GUN

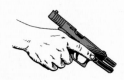

1: ALWAYS treat every firearm as if it were loaded. No ifs, ands, or buts. Even if you know the gun is unloaded, handle it as if it were loaded.

2: ALWAYS keep the firearm pointed in a safe direction, where a negligent discharge would cause minimum property damage and zero physical injury.

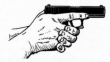

3: ALWAYS keep your trigger finger off the trigger and outside the trigger guard until you have made a conscious decision to shoot.

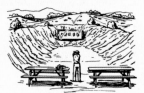

4: ALWAYS be sure of your target, backstop, and beyond. You must be aware of what's in your line of fire. This isn't usually a concern if you go to a professional gun range, but is a major concern when you go shoot with your buddy out on your property.

HOW TO FIRE A HANDGUN

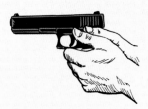

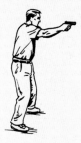

1: HOLD the handgun correctly. The gun hand (your dominant hand) should grip the gun high on the back strap (the back of the grip on the gun). Place your support (non-dominant) hand so that it is pressed firmly against the exposed portion of the grip not covered by the gun hand. All four fingers of your support hand should be under the trigger guard with the index finger pressed hard underneath it.

As you did with your gun hand, place your support hand as high as possible on the grip with the thumb pointing forward, roughly below where the slide meets the frame. Look at the back of your hands. There should be a distinct fit, like a puzzle, with your gun and support hand.

2: ASSUME the proper stance. Stand with your feet and hips shoulder-width apart. Bend your knees slightly. This "athletic stance" allows you to fire the weapon with stability and mobility. Raise the weapon toward your target.

Seek safety training from a real professional before pulling the trigger.

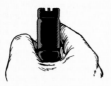

3: ALIGN your sights. Your handgun has a front sight and a rear sight notch. Aim at your target and align the top of the front sight with the top of the rear sight. There should also be equal amounts of empty space on both sides of the front sight.

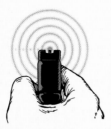

4: SET your sight picture. The sight picture is the pattern of your gun's sights in relation to your target. When you're aiming a gun, you're looking at three objects: the front sight, the rear sight, and your target. However, it's not possible to focus simultaneously on all three. One will inevitably be blurry when you're aiming. When you

have a correct sight picture, your front and rear sight appear sharp and clear and your target appears to be a bit blurry.

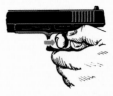

5: PRESS the trigger. Instead of pulling the trigger, squeeze the trigger straight to the rear. Apply constant, increasing pressure on the trigger until the weapon fires. Ensure that you're only applying pressure to the front of the trigger and not the sides.

ESCAPE DUCT TAPE RESTRAINTS

The power of duct tape cannot be overestimated. Whether it's holding on loose mufflers, patching holes in boats, or binding your hands after you've been kidnapped, this sticky stuff is the go-to tape to keep things in control. But if you find yourself with wrists bound up in man's favorite tool, know that trying to wriggle, writhe, or bite your way out will only leave you frustrated. For quick and easy freedom, follow this simple method.

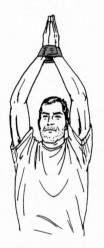

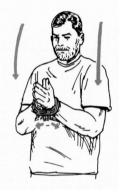

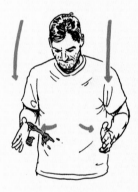

1: RAISE your hands high above your head.

2: PULL your arms down as quickly as possible, separating your hands as they contact your torso.

3: REPEAT as necessary until the duct tape splits and separates.

WALK LIKE A NINJA

Knowing how to walk stealthily is a useful skill, allowing you plan sneak attacks on your archenemies, steal cookies from coworkers, and check if toddlers are asleep without waking them.

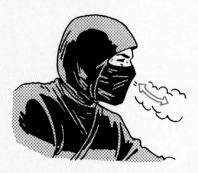

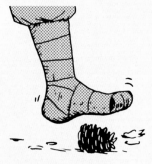

1: YOU'LL be tempted to hold your breath as you creep around. Don't. It will lead to loud and harsh exhales. Breathe slowly and calmly through the nose.

2: AS you vigilantly scan your surroundings, be sure to watch where you step. Watch for sticks, pinecones, and crunchy leaves outdoors, and toys, shoes, and table corners indoors.

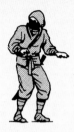

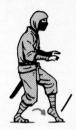

3: LOWER body for better balance and keep legs shoulder-width apart. Extend arms at waist level. Don't move your waist at all, just your legs.

4: START moving by balancing all your weight on your right leg. Move left foot forward, placing it lightly on the surface.

Toes and Ball of Foot First

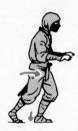

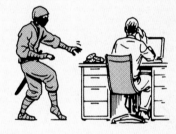

5: PUT your left heel down lightly. Slowly shift your body weight toward the ball of the left foot by bending your left knee and slowly leaning forward.

6: WITH your body weight supported by the ball of your left foot, slowly advance your right foot forward as you did in the last step. Repeat until you reach your target.

THE WARRIOR COLOR CODE

In life-or-death situations, psychological stress can get a man killed. To ensure you don't freeze or fail in an emergency, learn how to manage extreme stress. This code is used by soldiers, police officers, and first responders to assess preparedness in life-or-death situations.

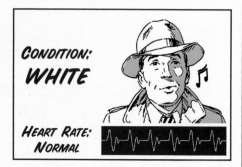

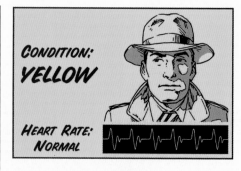

Condition White

YOU'RE UNAWARE of your surroundings and would be caught off-guard by a threat. The only time to be in Condition White is when you're secure at home or asleep.

Condition Yellow

THERE'S NO specific threat, and you're taking in your surroundings in a relaxed, but alert manner. Many Air Force pilots stick a yellow dot on their watch to remind them to stay in this state.

To manage stress effectively, you need to know what happens to your body in stressful situations.

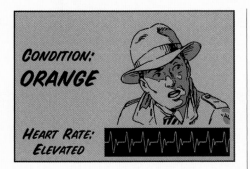

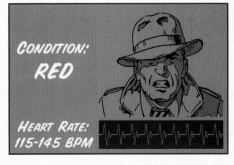

Condition Orange

YOU'VE IDENTIFIED a possible specific threat. Your goal isn't to take action, but to determine if it needs a response. Make a plan for what to do if you verify the threat. Stress levels and heart rate increase, but you experience no cognitive or motor deterioration.

Condition Red

YOU'VE VERIFIED the threat and are putting your plan into action. Adrenaline pumps through your veins and your heart rate is 115–145 beats per minute. This is the optimal level for tactical and survival scenarios. Complex motor skills and visual and cognitive reaction times are at their peak. Fine motor skills, like writing or threading flex cuffs, deteriorate.

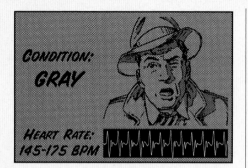

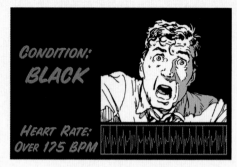

Condition Gray

YOUR HEART rate rises above the optimal range to reach 145–175 bpm. Tunnel vision, loss of depth perception, and auditory exclusion are common, which means you risk missing other threats or innocent bystanders. Complex motor skills—like gun manipulation—suffer, but gross motor skills—like running, jumping, pulling, and pushing—remain optimal.

Condition Black

YOUR HEART is beating faster than 175 bpm. Even well-trained fighters experience catastrophic breakdown of performance at this level. In addition to the symptoms of Condition Gray, you may void your bladder and bowels. In anonymous surveys conducted after WWII, one-quarter of soldiers admitted they peed themselves and one-eighth admitted to defecating during combat. Blood vessels narrow to constrict blood flow, which deteriorates complex motor skills. Your forebrain shuts down and your primitive middle brain takes over, making you susceptible to irrational fighting, fleeing, or freezing.

DEVELOP SITUATIONAL AWARENESS

Situational awareness is knowing what's going on around you. It sounds easy, but it requires much practice. And while it is taught to soldiers and law enforcement officers, it's an important skill for civilians as well. In a dangerous situation, being aware of a threat even seconds before everyone else can keep you and your loved ones safe.

HOW TO DEVELOP SITUATIONAL AWARENESS

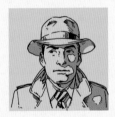

Stay in Condition Yellow

FOR OPTIMAL situational awareness, stay in Condition Yellow of Cooper's Color Code (see page 166): "relaxed alert." There's no specific threat, but you're taking in your surroundings with all your senses. Even though your senses are heightened, stay relaxed. Adopting a calm demeanor won't attract unnecessary attention. Don't zone out: look up from your smartphone, open your eyes, ears, and nose, and calmly scan your environment to take it in.

Establish Baselines, Anomalies, and Action Plans

BEING MORE observant isn't enough to master situational awareness. You have to know what you're looking for, and put that information into context so it has meaning and becomes actionable. We do that by establishing baselines, anomalies, and action plans.

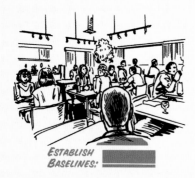

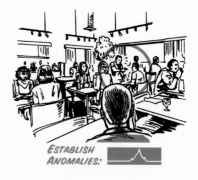

Establish a Baseline Wherever You Go

A BASELINE is what's "normal" in a given situation, and differs from person to person and environment to environment. The baseline at a small coffee shop will usually entail people reading books or working on their computers or speaking in hushed tones with friends. The baseline at a rock concert would be loud music and people looking at the stage while jumping up and down to the music or swaying to the beat.

Establish Anomalies

WE ESTABLISH baselines so that we can spot anomalies. According to Patrick Van Horne, situational awareness expert, instructor of the Marine Combat Profiling system, and author of Left of Bang, "Anomalies are things that either do not happen and should, or that do happen and shouldn't."

Know what to look for in order to act.

WE ESTABLISH baselines so that we can direct our attention to anomalies. How do we do that on the fly? Mentally ask yourself these questions when you enter a new environment:

- Baseline Questions: What's going on here? What's the general mood of the place? What's the "normal" activity that I should expect here? How do most people behave here most of the time?
- Anomaly Question: What would cause someone or something to stand out?

IMPORTANT ANOMALIES to look out for involve conscious and subconscious body language. Of particular note for situational awareness are dominance/submissive, comfortable/uncomfortable, and interested/uninterested behaviors.

DOMINANT/SUBMISSIVE BEHAVIOR.
Most people try to get along with others, so they act in accommodating and submissive ways. Dominant behavior thus constitutes an anomaly, and the person displaying it deserves more attention. If someone acts pushy, authoritative, or overbearing, it doesn't necessarily mean they're a threat; context matters. You'd expect bosses to act dominant in relation to their employees and the employees to act submissive to their boss, but a customer exhibiting extreme dominant behavior toward an employee isn't as common. Keep an eye on it.

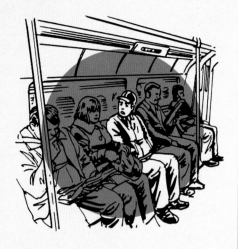

COMFORTABLE/UNCOMFORTABLE BE-HAVIOR. Most people look relatively comfortable in most situations. Think about a bus ride—passengers appear generally relaxed while they stare out the window or read a book. If someone looks uncomfortable, that warrants extra attention, but they may not be a threat. They could be distressed because they're late for work or heard bad news about a relative. Again, keep an eye on it.

A COMMON display of uncomfortable behavior you'll see from individuals up to no good is "checking their six": looking over their shoulder behind them or scanning their surroundings. Most people don't do this because they don't feel any threat. If a guy looks over his shoulder a lot when he should be standing aloof, that warrants your attention.

OF COURSE, "checking your six" is something that situationally aware good guys do too. If you're doing it right, it shouldn't be noticeable to others, but that takes practice, and the guy with his head on a swivel might still be green. But until you verify that through observation, be suspicious.

ON THE flip side, someone acting comfortable when everyone else is uncomfortable is also an anomaly. One of the ways law enforcement identified the Boston Marathon bombers was by noticing in surveillance footage that the men looked relatively calm while everyone else was in a panic. They knew the explosions were going to happen, while everyone else was caught off guard.

INTERESTED/UNINTERESTED BEHAVIOR. Most people aren't paying attention to their environment. They're too caught up in their own thoughts or what they're doing. So individuals showing interest in a particular person or object that most people wouldn't be interested in are anomalies that warrant observation.

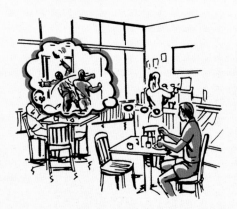

Create a Plan of Action

1: ONCE you've answered the baseline and anomaly questions, ask yourself a third question: "What would I do if I saw an anomaly?" In other words, come up with an action plan.

2: LET'S say you're in a coffee shop and the anomaly for which you want to create an action plan is "guy comes in with a gun." The best course of action will depend on a few things—and knowing those things requires you to be situationally aware. If the robber came in from the front and you're near the rear exit, your best action would be to book it out the back door right away. On the other hand, if he entered through the back exit near you, your best action might be to immediately close the gap and incapacitate him.

3: ESTABLISH baselines. Look for anomalies. Have a plan. That's situational awareness.

MANAGE STRESS
IN HIGH STAKES SITUATIONS

You can't completely control your heart rate in a high-stress situation, but you can maximize your resistance to stress to perform at optimal levels (i.e., stay in Condition Red) for as long as possible.

We don't rise to the level of our expectations,
we fall to the level of our training.

—Archilochus

1: PRACTICE tactical breathing, a technique that soldiers and police officers use to calm down and stay focused during firefights: Slowly inhale a deep breath for four seconds. Hold the breath in for four seconds. Slowly exhale the breath for four seconds. Hold the empty breath for four seconds. Then repeat until your breathing is under control.

2: MEDITATE. Meditation can help clear stressful thoughts from your mind. To meditate, sit in a quiet place and focus on your breath going in your nose and out your mouth. When a distracting thought pops up, name the thought, let it go, and focus back on your breath. With time your mind will quiet down, and your ability to dismiss unwanted thoughts will improve. Start with one ten-minute session daily, and slowly increase to twenty minutes.

3: PRACTICE visualization. Warriors who visualize hypothetical high-stress scenarios perform better in actual situations than those who don't.

- Make the visualization as vivid as possible. Incorporate your senses and emotions.
- Visualize yourself successfully overcoming specific obstacles. Never visualize failure.
- Combine visualization with tactical practice and role playing.

4: USE task-relevant instructional self-talk. To counter the effects of high stress, talk yourself through complex actions as if you were an instructor. For example, many police officers are trained to speak out loud during every step in the gun firing process using the acronym BRASS: Breathe, Relax, Aim, Sight, Squeeze.

5: TRAIN realistically. There's an old saying among soldiers: "You do not rise to the occasion in combat, you sink to the level of training." For self-defense, do more than go to the gun range or punch a heavy bag. Train under the same pressure you'll experience in real life. This can be achieved with simunitions or airsoft guns, or live sparring.

ACTIVE SHOOTER TRIAGE

According to the FBI, active shootings in public places are becoming increasingly common. Instead of focusing on the political debate these events create, we'll discuss what you can actually do in these unlikely situations. Most active shootings end in two minutes or less. That's not enough time for law enforcement to arrive. If you hear gunshots, you won't have much time to act.

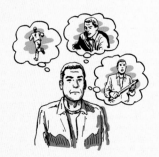

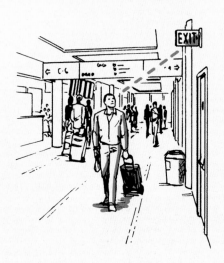

1: WHEN emergency strikes, the natural response for most people is to do nothing. When we see others cowering in fear, we tend to act the same way. The way to overcome passivity is to know what you'll do in the event of a shooting before one ever happens. To act on that plan, you must maintain situational awareness. Stay in condition yellow, or "relaxed alert," establishing baselines of what's normal, looking for aberrations, and staying aware of exits.

2: WHEN you've heard shots and screams, what should you do? Experts agree that you have three options: run, hide, and fight—in that order.

RUN

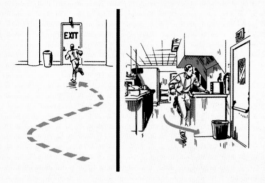

1: AS soon as you hear gunfire, leave the premises immediately using your escape plan, and get as far away from the shooter as possible, without crossing the shooter's path. As you exit, tell others to come along. Once out of danger, call 911—don't assume someone else will.

2: KEEP your hands visible so law enforcement can see you are not a threat, and don't try to assist the wounded while making your exit. Even the first law enforcement officers to arrive at the scene will initially ignore the wounded so they can take out the shooter. Your top priority is to get to safety.

3: IF you're in an open area with distance between you and the shooter, run as fast as you can in a zig-zag pattern, taking cover behind barriers that can stop bullets. Shooting a moving target is hard even for experienced marksmen, and many mass shooters have little experience with firearms.

HIDE

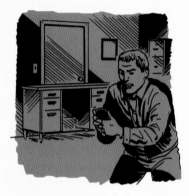

1: SOMETIMES running isn't an option. The next best thing is to hide in a secure location out of the shooter's view in a place that can provide protection from gunfire. If you're in an office or school building, find a room with a lockable door. If you can't lock the door, barricade it. He's often looking for easy victims and may move on rather than push through the barrier. Stay away from the door and crouch behind items that could offer protection from bullets, like cabinets or desks. Hide in a bathroom or closet if you can.

2: TURN off the lights and be as quiet as possible. Put your cell phone on silent—you don't even want it on vibrate. If possible, dial 911 and let the authorities know there's an active shooter in your building. If you can't speak because the shooter is nearby, leave the line open so the dispatcher can hear what's going on.

3: DON'T open the door unless you can confirm the authorities are knocking. Shooters may yell for help in the hopes of convincing people to show themselves.

4: IF you can't find a room in which to secure yourself, hide in a location that offers cover and concealment from the shooter, but still allows you to see him. If the shooter passes you, you can make a run for it. If he doesn't, it puts you in a position to attack if necessary.

Run, Hide, and Fight —In That Order

FIGHT

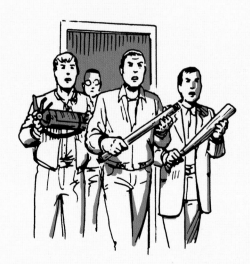

1: WHEN running or hiding have failed or aren't viable options, you may have to resort to plan C: Fight. Even if you don't carry a firearm, commit to the idea that if you absolutely have to (and, again, we're talking the very last resort here), you'll attack quickly and devastatingly.

FIGHT AN ACTIVE SHOOTER

As a last resort after running or hiding, you may need to fight for your life in an active shooter scenario.

If you're armed, there are techniques you should employ in returning fire. A tutorial on how to take down a gunman lies outside the purview of this book, and must be practiced in the real world with trained professionals. If you're not armed, real world practice in hand-to-hand fighting will be an enormous asset, giving you concrete skills to employ and a greater comfort level with violence and confidence in taking action.

But if you're the most average of average joes, with neither a gun nor a black belt, you can still attempt to take on a gunman as a last resort.

1: KNOW your advantages. Most violent gunmen work under the assumption that people will do what they want or hide. By doing the unexpected (attacking), you're disrupting the gunman's OODA Loop (the Observe, Orient, Decide, and Act cycle on page 232), which slows him down—even for just a few seconds—and gives you more time to win the battle.

2: A gun can only be shot in one direction at any one time. If you approach the shooter from behind or from the side, it's going to be harder to shoot you. What's more, if you attack the shooter as a team (which you should), he can't shoot everyone at the same time. An attack by multiple people, from multiple angles, will be difficult for a lone gunman to fend off.

3: BE aggressive and violent. This isn't the time for pussyfooting. Attack with violence and aggression. Use lethal force, and don't stop fighting until the shooter stops moving.

4: CONTROL the weapon and then control the shooter. The sooner you can get the weapon out of the shooter's hands, without endangering others, the better. Once the weapon has been secured, turn your attention to containing the perpetrator. Sometimes you're not going to be in a position to secure the weapon first, so your priority would be to inflict as much violence as possible on the shooter until you can get the gun away.

5: IF you can't get the gun out of the attacker's hands, do what you can to control it. If the shooter has a semi-automatic pistol, grab the barrel as hard as you can. You can control where it's pointed, and if the gun does fire, this will prevent the slide from chambering a new round.

6: USE improvised weapons. Look for chairs, fire extinguishers, umbrellas, belts, coffee mugs. Even a pen can multiply the impact of your force. Throw stuff at the shooter. Even if it doesn't disable him, you're creating hesitation, which will give you more time to end the fight. Use items to blind the shooter: Flash a high-beam flashlight in his eyes, spray a fire extinguisher in his face, or throw a pot of hot coffee his way. Once the shooter is disoriented, rush him and take him down.

7: WORK as a team. The more people you can get to help you in attacking the shooter, the better your chances of ending the ordeal with few casualties. Most people's natural reaction is not to do anything. Be assertive and take the lead. Courage is contagious.

A gun can only be shot in one direction at any one time.

DEFEND YOURSELF FROM A KNIFE ATTACK

It's been said to "never bring a knife to a gun fight." Whoever said that has never been at the receiving end of a knife attack. Knives require little skill to use effectively, and knife assailants rarely miss their target. If you're surprised by a knife attack, you may have no chance to react. But if you know someone is coming after you, here's how to increase your chance of surviving an attack.

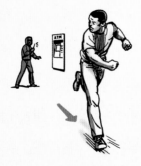

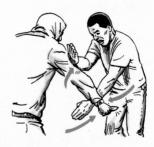

1: RUN away. Seriously. As soon as you see the glint of a steel knife, turn and run as fast as you can. You're better off outpacing your attacker than trying to Bruce Lee the knife away from him. In the process of defending yourself, you'll likely be slashed, gashed, or stabbed even if you do survive.

2: USE the "Split-X" Block. If running isn't an option, your goal is to keep the knife from sticking and slashing you. Most knife attackers use a forward thrust technique because it's simple and effective. One way to block this attack is the "Split X." As the assailant's attack arm comes toward you, drop your hands and make an "X" with your arms. Simultaneously, throw your hips back. The assailant's arm will hit the apex of your arms and prevent the knife from hitting you.

A knife attack is a nasty, dangerous affair. The best thing you can do when you see the glint of steel is to get as far away from your attacker as possible.

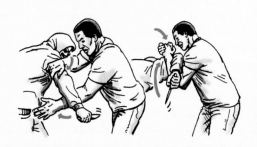

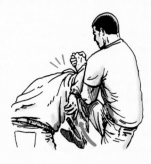

3: CONTROL his arm. As soon as you block the assailant's arm, take control of it. Use the top hand in your "Split X" to grab his arm. Bring your bottom hand up and clasp your top hand firmly. Using your clasped hands as leverage, squeeze your arms together, smashing your assailant's arm in between your forearms.

4: VIOLENTLY knee assailant in face. In this arm hold position, your attacker's face is in perfect alignment for a good face kneeing. Violently knee him in the face until he drops the knife.

ESCAPE ZIP TIE HANDCUFFS

Standard zip ties from the hardware store are increasingly being used to restrain innocent people in home invasion and kidnapping scenarios. Thankfully, with a little practice and the right technique, you can escape from zip ties. We tried out all of these methods, and they all work—even with the heaviest-duty variety, rated at 175 pounds.

SLIPPING OUT

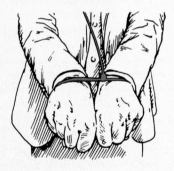

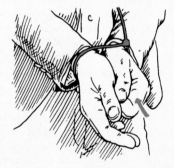

1: PRESENT your hands to your captor with fists clenched and palms facing down. Doing this makes your wrist bigger and creates room to slip out.

2: AFTER the tie is tightened, unclench, turn your wrists so they're facing inward, and work your way out. It may be tight, but the key is to just get your thumb out first. This method can be used from a variety of hand positions, and should be tried first.

BREAKING ZIP TIES

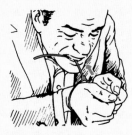 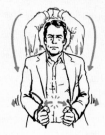 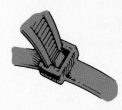

1: TIGHTEN zip ties as much as you can with your teeth and try to make sure the locking mechanism is between your hands. The tighter the zip tie, the easier it is to break.

2: LIFT hands above head and bring them down quickly into your stomach. Your elbows should flare out like chicken wings, and you should simulate trying to touch your shoulder blades together. With that, the ties should break at their weakest point—the locking mechanism.

SHIMMING OUT

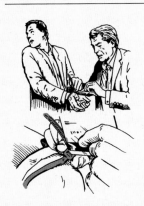

1: DEFEAT the mechanism of the zip tie with some kind of shim. If you look closely at a zip tie, you'll see it has a small locking bar that does all the work. If that bar is lifted from the tracks of the zip tie, it can be easily removed.

2: YOU can use a variety of objects to lift that locking bar: a fingernail, a pin, even a credit card. Once the bar is lifted, simply pull the tie out of the locking mechanism. This method is easier with multiple people held captive to help each other, but can be done on your own.

ESCAPE FROM THE TRUNK OF A CAR

The trunk of a car is nothing more than a mobile prison. Locked up and on the move, your window of escape may not last long. Time your escape at an opportune moment, when you suspect the car is without occupants or traveling slowly; popping out of the trunk while cruising down the highway at speed wouldn't be an improvement to your situation. Act quietly and quickly at the right moment and you may escape successfully.

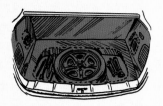

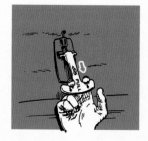

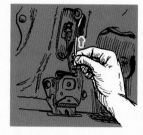

1: SEARCH for tools that might help you escape. Compartments under the trunk's floor may hold flashlights, pry bars, and other hand tools.

2: PULL the trunk release handle found on most modern cars. It's usually glow-in-the-dark and located near the center of the trunk lid.

3: FIND and pull the cable that runs from the trunk to the trunk release lever near the driver. Search the driver's side of the trunk and pull the cable toward the front of the car.

The trunk of a car is nothing more than a mobile prison.

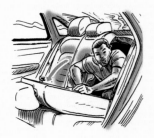

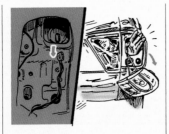

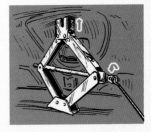

4: TRY forcing your way through the backseat by pulling a seat release cable or kicking at the seat.

5: KICK out the brake light to create a hole through which you can signal to other drivers for help.

6: USE a car jack, if you can find one, to force the trunk lid open enough to escape or signal for help.

Chapter 5

The
FAMILY MAN

There is no doubt that it is around the family and the home that all the greatest virtues, the most dominating virtues of human society, are created, strengthened, and maintained.

—Winston Churchill

FAMILY IS the laboratory of our lives. Within our families we learn and practice all the vital skills of human flourishing. From your father, you may have learned how to handle a hammer; from your mother, how to cook a killer roast. And from constant interactions with your parents and siblings you gain an education in how to love, reconcile, sacrifice, and compromise.

No matter your age or station in life, you have a role to play as a Family Man. If you're a son, you have the filial duty to look after your parents. If you're a father, you have the responsibility to create a family culture that will help your children grow into virtuous and capable adults. If you're an uncle, you have the sacred charge of teaching your nieces and nephews all the dangerous stuff their mother or father won't let them do at home. And if you're married, you are a confidant and support to your partner. If you're all of these things, your responsibilities and privileges extend up, down, and across your family tree. You're a fortunate man.

COMMANDMENTS OF CLEAN COMMUNICATION

Loving relationships are the most important contributor to a man's happiness, success, and ability to live a fully flourishing life.

One of the most important factors in creating and sustaining these relationships is communication. Unfortunately, how to communicate with one's significant other in a healthy, positive way is something we are rarely taught. As a result, many couples find that their discussions regularly turn into unproductive arguments that damage their bond.

Couples who discuss their disagreements in a healthy way are able to solve problems before they turn into big, relationship-ending issues. Here are a few guidelines to follow as you talk to your loved one to handle disagreements effectively and cleanly.

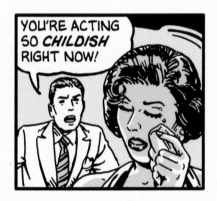

1: **AVOID** judgment words or loaded terms.

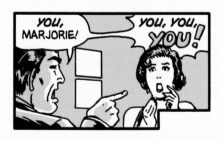

2: AVOID "you" messages of blame and accusation.

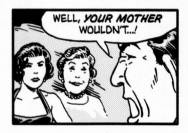

4: AVOID negative comparisons.

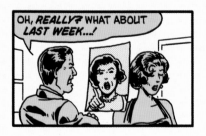

3: DON'T rehash old history.

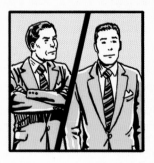

5: KEEP body language open and receptive.

KEEP A TREASURE BOX

The ditty-box is a timeless tradition that every man should have. It's a great way to store your memories as well as those small assortments you use on a regular basis like tie bars and watches. Someday your kids will enjoy rummaging through your manly treasures and hearing the stories behind the interesting things you've picked up along life's way!

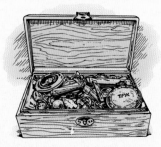

We used to wait in the library in the evening until we could hear his key rattling in the latch of the front hall, and then rush out to greet him; and we would troop into his room while he was dressing, to stay there as long as we were permitted, eagerly examining anything which came out of his pockets which could be regarded as an attractive novelty. Every child has fixed in his memory various details which strike it as of grave importance. The trinkets he used to keep in a little box on his dressing-table we children always used to speak of as "treasures." The word, and some of the trinkets themselves, passed on to the next generation. My own children, when small, used to troop into my room while I was dressing, and the gradually accumulating trinkets in the "ditty-box"— the gift of an enlisted man in the navy—always excited rapturous joy.

—Theodore Roosevelt

DELIVER A BABY

Don't get all clammy: A man caught in the tight situation of having to help with an unexpected birth won't actually need to do much. In fact, your greatest role in delivering a child is enabling the natural process of birth to run its course. Provide a calm, clean, and safe environment for the mother and wait for trained medical help to do the rest.

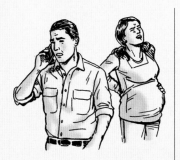

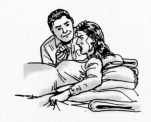

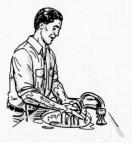

1: CALL for help. Dial 911 and have an ambulance sent to your location. The dispatcher may also be able to offer you instructions and guide you through the next steps.

2: PREPARE a birthing area by laying down clean sheets and collecting plenty of clean, dry towels. Natural birthing positions for the mother are lying on her back, or with her hands and knees on the ground.

3: THOROUGHLY wash your hands and arms up to the elbow to avoid spreading germs and other contaminants to the baby once it's born.

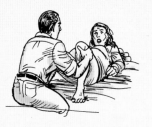

4: FOLLOW the woman's lead. As she feels the urge to push, encourage her. You should be able to see the baby's head beginning to exit the birth canal. If you see the umbilical cord is wrapped around the baby's neck, gently loosen it.

Never pull on the baby or try to force it out.

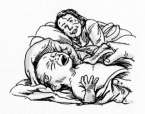

5: DRY the baby with clean towels once it's born, wipe away any gunk in the nose, eyes, and mouth, and keep it warm. Place the baby onto the mother's chest.

Do not cut the umbilical cord.

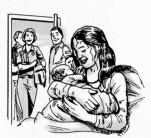

6: APPROX. 15–30 minutes after the birth, the mother will pass the placenta. Deliver the placenta if medical help hasn't arrived. Wait calmly for paramedics to arrive, and give yourself a pat on the back!

HOLD A BABY

There is a lot to fatherhood that you have to learn from trial and error. But honing your skill set before your progeny arrives can help the experience of being a new dad go more smoothly. With all of the baby-handling tips outlined in the next several pages, don't worry so much about hurting your baby. They're not as fragile as you think. Sturdy little buggers, really.

Holding your baby skin-to-skin can calm and comfort him—stabilizing his heart rate, respiratory rate, and blood pressure, maintaining his body temperature, and decreasing his crying. It also helps you bond. Soon after your baby is born, and for the next few weeks, spend time with your shirt off holding him just in his diaper.

Whatever hold you use, the important thing is to support your baby's neck, bottom, and small of the back.

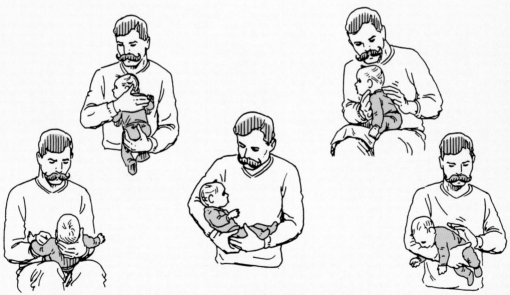

BURP A BABY

Babies get gas from sucking in air while feeding. Burping helps get these air bubbles out. If you're feeding a baby with a bottle, burp her after every 2–3 ounces she drinks, as well as at the end of her feeding. If she's fussy or spits up a lot, try burping even more often during the feeding. With all of these methods, give your baby gentle pats or small, circular rubs to get the burp out.

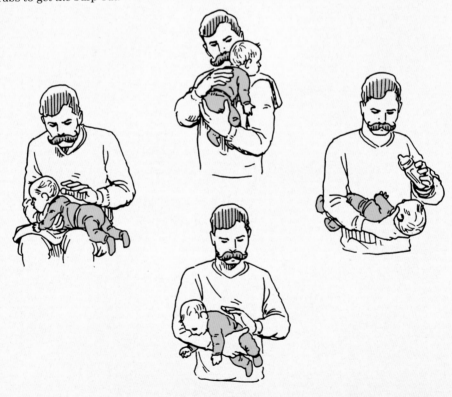

CHANGE A DIAPER

Spread the diaper in the position of the [baseball] diamond with you at bat.
Then fold second base down to home and set the baby on the pitcher's mound. Put
first base and third together, bring up home plate, and pin the three together. Of
course, in case of rain, you gotta call the game and start all over again.

—Jimmy Piersall, MLB center fielder

A new baby is a poop and pee machine. You'll be amazed that such a small person can produce so much waste. You can expect to change a newborn's diaper every two hours. Though science has yet to create a self-cleaning baby, the changings get less frequent as they get older.

1: ASSESS the damage. Be prepared for anything. You might have a little nugget waiting for you, or you could have a hazardous waste explosion. If the latter, move the baby near the bath, so you can thoroughly clean her.

2: GET your materials. Grab a clean diaper and four or five baby wipes (if it's #2). Place them to the side.

3: PUT your gas mask on and assume the position. If your baby is formula fed, be prepared for a potent smell. If your baby is breast-fed, the stink isn't quite as bad. If you have a boy, juke to the side lest his little sprinkler baptize you into the Church of the Yellow Stream.

4: UNDO the dirty diaper and lift up your baby's tuchus by grabbing her ankles and gently hoisting her feet into the air. Use a clean part of the dirty diaper to wipe excess poo from her behind.

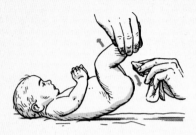

5: GRAB a baby wipe and start wiping front to back. This motion reduces the chance of spreading bacteria into their privates, which can cause a urinary tract infection (especially important for girls). Place the used wipes on top of the soiled diaper. Then, with your baby's feet still suspended in the air, remove the soiled diaper.

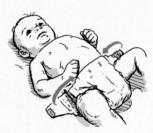

6: FOLD the diaper on itself with the hazardous waste and used wipes still in it. Use the sticky tabs to make a tight bundle. Place inside a plastic bag, tie the bag off, and hook shot the bundle into the diaper bin.

7: PAT your baby's bottom dry. Apply some A&D or Desitin if her butt is red or irritated.

8: SLIDE the new diaper under her. The back of the diaper has the sticky tabs on it. Lay your baby down on this part.

9: BRING up the front of the diaper and attach the tabs. You want it tight enough so that it doesn't slide off but not so tight it cuts off circulation. Most disposable diapers have little ruffles around the leg. Make sure those are sticking out, or you'll have some leaking problems.

10: GIVE your baby a high five.

CALM A CRYING BABY

The most important skill to have as a new dad (if you wish to maintain your sanity) is being able to calm your baby when he or she cries. Whether your baby cries a lot or a little will probably determine whether your parenting experience is easier or harder than you expected. Unfortunately, you can't choose whether you get a really happy baby or a cantankerous caterwauler. But there's usually a reason why your baby is crying; when something is bothering her, she doesn't have any way to communicate besides howling.

1: FIRST, run through a mental checklist of what could have put a bee in her bonnet:

- Dirty diaper: See page 197.

- Needs to burp: Try page 196.

- Gas: Lay her on her back and move her legs up and down like she's riding a bicycle, or gently massage her tummy in a circle. You can try over-the-counter remedies like simethicone and "gripe water"—but they don't work for everyone.

- Physical discomfort: Is she too hot or cold? Is clothing tight or scratchy?

- Loneliness: The world is a big, unfamiliar place. If she wakes up and no one is around, she might just want to be held.

- Overstimulation: Too much new stuff to take in all at once can make your baby feel overwhelmed. Take her somewhere quiet to decompress.

- Hunger: Feed her!

- Tired: Time for a nap.

- Fever: An easy-to-use forehead thermometer is a must. If she's running a temperature, you can give her some baby acetaminophen, but be sure to check with your doctor for the right dosage.

IF THE checklist doesn't work, you may have a case of undiagnosed crankiness. It happens to all of us. Try this:

2: STICK a pacifier in it. Not all babies take to the pacifier, and there are pros and cons to using one, but they can work wonders in silencing a newborn.

3: PUT the baby in a motorized swing. It works like a charm for some kids.

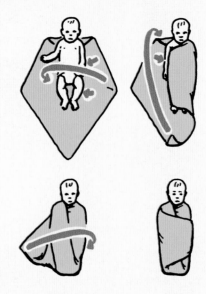

No matter how much a baby cries, stay as zen as possible.

4: SWADDLE. Babies like being tightly wrapped—it reminds them of being back in the womb.

5: RUN the vacuum. The womb was a surprisingly loud place, so replicate that white noise to put your baby at ease.

6: TAKE 'em for a drive. When all else fails, stick the baby in her car seat and take her for a drive.

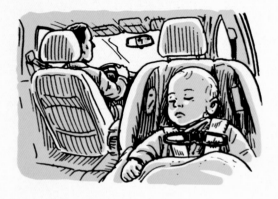

7: RECOGNIZE colic. If none of the above stops the caterwauling, and she cries for three hours a day for more than three days a week for three weeks, she may have colic. Its cause is unknown. Try the "5 S's" (Swaddle, Stomach/Side position, Shush, Swing, Suck) as proposed in *The Happiest Baby on the Block* and hang in there. It often resolves itself four to six months in.

8: KEEP calm. Babies' cries are designed by nature to burrow into your brain and elicit a real physiological response—you start to sweat, your heart rate goes up, and your body releases cortisol—the stress hormone. Deal with this the way you would any other stressor. It can be helpful to disassociate yourself from the cries—tell yourself that it's okay, it's just a noise. Practice your tactical breathing. If your brain is starting to short-circuit, there's nothing wrong with putting your baby down in a safe place like her crib, closing the door, going into another room where you can't hear her cries, and taking five. Your baby will be fine—really. It's better to let her cry for a little while than for you to lose control.

USE YOUR BABY AS EXERCISE EQUIPMENT

I t's hard to fit in a good workout as a new dad. But you may be surprised how many exercises you can perform using only your kiddo and a car seat. What's more, when you use your tot as a piece of exercise equipment, your little champ gets all the benefits that come with roughhousing.

Make sure you wait to do these exercises until your baby is ready for the action. Before you start tossing them around, they should be able to hold their neck up and sit up by themselves.

— BABY + KETTLEBELL —	— BABY + MEDICINE BALL —

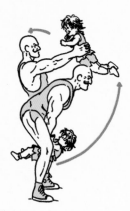

Baby Kettlebell Swing

*Hold baby by torso BELOW arms,
not BY the arms*

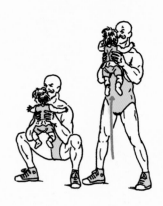

Baby Goblet Squat

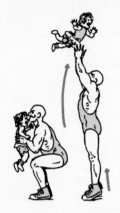

Baby Medicine Ball Toss

BABY + DUMBBELL

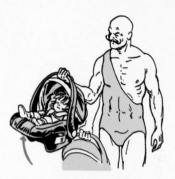

Baby Bicep Curls

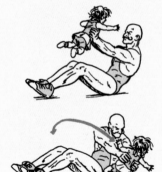

Baby Torso Rotation

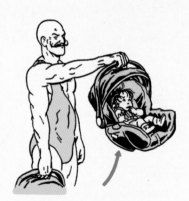

Baby Front Raises

BE SANTA CLAUS

If your family celebrates Christmas, and you're of the opinion that belief in Santa Claus constitutes one of the most magical parts of childhood rather than the Big Lie, you'll have the privilege of taking on the role of old Kris Kringle. This is a big responsibility. For eight or so years of your kids' lives, you'll be playing the jolly old fat man who makes dreams come true. If you do it well, your kids' imaginations will have plenty of magical moments to feast on. If you blow it, your kids may become prematurely jaded about Christmas.

BEING SANTA is no easy task; kids today are savvy, and the truth about Mr. Claus is only a Google search away. Here's how to preserve the Christmas magic and keep your kids believing in St. Nick for as long as possible.

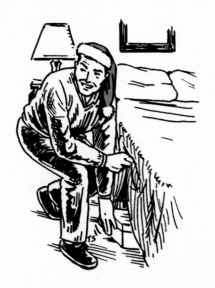

1: HIDE the gifts. The most common Santa slayer for kids is finding the gifts that are supposedly being made in Santa's workshop sitting in their parents' closet. Around age six or seven kids start getting suspicious about the Santa story and will commence a thorough search of the house to find their Christmas booty. These are professional hide-n-seekers, so don't fool yourself: they know every nook and cranny. If you don't have a super-secret spot available in-residence, stash the presents offsite—at your office, if you have space, or at the house of a friend who 1) has no kids, 2) has infants, or 3) has older kids who are in on the Santa jig.

2: TRACK Santa on radar. Little tykes now look to modern gadgets for affirmation of what is real. Every year NORAD radar realistically "tracks" Santa's journey around the globe on Christmas Eve. You can show this to your kids as proof that Santa is indeed on the move.

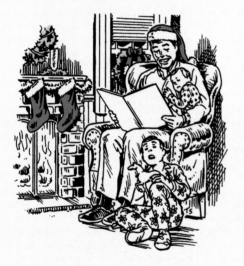

3: GET the kids to bed. Read the kiddos The Night Before Christmas and/or The Polar Express and then tuck them into bed. But they're going to have a tough time getting to sleep; kids are wired on Christ-mas Eve night, excitedly thinking about all the cool stuff that they're going to get in the morning. To make sure they actually doze off so you and your wife can get to work, tell them that Santa Claus has a sleep detector and will only come to homes that have sleeping children. If that doesn't work, give them a sippy cup filled with eggnog and a bit of rum.

We're just kidding about the eggnog and rum in a sippy cup.

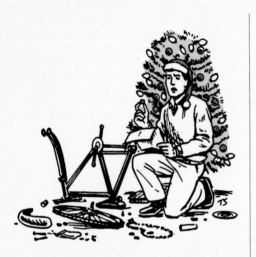

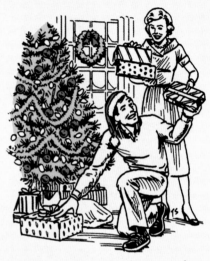

4: FINISH assembling toys. Some presents, like bikes, will need some assembly. If possible, do any assembly offsite in order to reduce the ruckus of you going through your toolbox. If that's not an option, get the tools you need ready during the day. Read the instructions so you have an idea of what you're doing. You have limited time, so the less time you spend scratching your head figuring out how to put the darn thing together the better.

5: PLACE the presents under the tree and fill the stockings. If possible, wrap all the presents before Christmas Eve so all you have to do that night is put them under the tree. While you or your wife bring out the gifts, the other stuffs the stockings with goodies. Pro tip: In the run up to Christmas, remember to hide the stocking goodies as well as you hide the big presents.

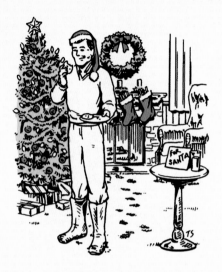

6: AS you put out the presents, be on watch for rogue children. Kids will invariably climb out of bed to either try to sneak a peek at Santa Claus himself or see if he's left their booty under the tree yet. If at all possible, try to catch your kids before they make it near the living area where the tree and gifts are waiting. Threaten them with a lump of coal if they don't get back to bed. If you can't stop your kid in time and he catches you in the act, you can lie and

maintain their faith in Santa or tell them the sad truth that Santa isn't real. If you go with the more fun option, i.e., lying, tell your kid that you and your wife were just putting out Mommy's and Daddy's gifts for each other and that Santa had already come. Swiftly get them back to bed so you can finish the job.

7: LEAVE evidence. Unlike most men who sneak into houses late at night, Santa leaves plenty of evidence behind. Leave some sooty boot prints on the carpet near the fireplace. Eat the milk and cookies, leaving some half-eaten cookies on the plate. If the kids set out carrots for the reindeer, put some gnawed-on carrot stubs in the fireplace. Maybe place a cool gold button near the Christmas tree, too, and tell your kids that it must have fallen off Santa's suit.

8: GET to bed. You won't get much sleep tonight, but try to get as much shuteye as you can. You're going to need all the energy you can get on Christmas Day.

ENTERTAIN A TODDLER
WITHOUT A SMARTPHONE

Our smartphones allow us to do many things more efficiently, they entertain us when we're bored, and they keep us informed when we need answers. But life's most rewarding activities are analog. As younger generations wade into a world filled with technology, it's important to give them a good foundation of old-fashioned fun. The next time you're in charge of engaging the attention of a kid, don't turn to silly videos and games on your phone. Instead, show them how to have a great time, tech-free.

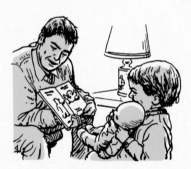

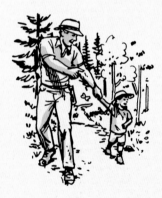

1: READ a book, making sure you do voices for different characters with maximum enthusiasm.

2: GO on a nature walk to teach them about basic plants and look for bugs.

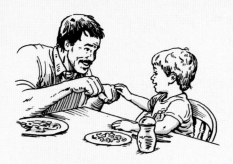

3: PLAY a game like "Guess Which Hand," where you have them place an object in one of your hands, close your fists, put your hands behind your back, switch the object around, and then have them guess which hand the object is in.

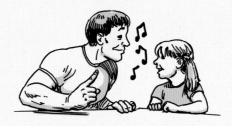

4: TEACH them a simple song like "Twinkle Twinkle, Little Star," "Old MacDonald," or "Baa Baa Black Sheep."

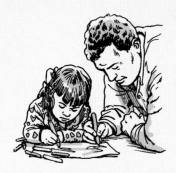

5: PRACTICE drawing with colored pencils, washable markers, or sidewalk chalk and teach them to make basic shapes and figures.

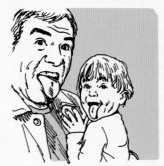

6: MAKE faces and noises at each other to see who can be sillier.

TREAT YOUR FAMILY LIKE VIPS

Even if you don't work as a personal security agent, if you're a man with a family, you've got VIPs you're responsible for keeping safe: your wife and kiddos.

WHILE YOU may not have the resources to do the same sort of preparation as a professional personal security detail, you can apply the same ethos when taking care of your family.

———— BE THOUGHTFUL ABOUT YOUR EDC ————
(EVERY DAY CARRY)

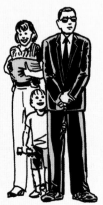
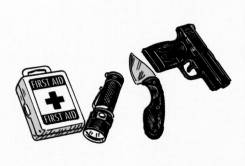

ALWAYS HAVE a first aid kit in your car for minor injuries, and keep tourniquets in the kit to stop bleeding in the event of an active shooting or similar attack. On your person, keep at a minimum your cell phone (to call emergency crews) and a tactical flashlight. A bright flashlight helps identify threats in the dark and can momentarily disorient attackers. It doubles as an improvised weapon.

CONSIDER CARRYING A WEAPON

WHETHER TO carry weapons to defend your family is a decision only you can make. If you do decide to carry a firearm, understand the laws governing its use in self-defense and train regularly with it. Carrying a gun without knowing how to use it and regularly practicing your marksmanship is dangerous. If you don't want to carry a firearm, or you live somewhere that doesn't allow it, you can carry a knife (though some localities also forbid this). If you don't want to carry a weapon, carry a

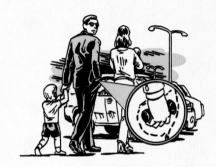

tactical pen that can improvise as a weapon if needed. You can bring it anywhere discreetly and legally.

IF A PLACE LOOKS LIKE TROUBLE, LEAVE

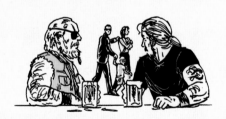

THE BEST outcome for a personal security agent is if the principal never encounters the potential for harm, harassment, or embarrassment. That's your job, too. When you're out with your family, survey the place you're in. Be prepared to leave if you don't think it's safe. Don't be paranoid, but don't let inconvenience deter you from protecting your family.

MAINTAIN SITUATIONAL AWARENESS

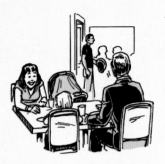

PUT YOURSELF in a position of optimal observance. At a restaurant, ask to be seated at a table with the best vantage point. You want to see as many exits and entrances as possible.

ESTABLISH BASELINES and look for anomalies. Hands hold what can kill you; faces (particularly eyes) show intent. Don't stare people down one by one. Just play it cool, glance at hands and faces, and actually notice what you see. And remember: An anomaly isn't necessarily a threat.

HAVE A plan. In every place you go, make a plan for what you'll do if you notice an anomaly. What would you do if someone entered the theater through an emergency exit? It could be a kid trying to sneak in for a free movie, or it could be an active shooter. Increase your level of alertness and decide what you'll do should the interloper turn violent.

IF SOMEONE IS GIVING YOUR FAMILY TROUBLE, LEAVE. DON'T ESCALATE.

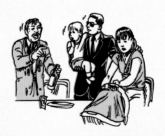

IF YOUR family is facing an imminent, life-threatening attack, your priority is to keep them safe. That usually means getting them out as fast as possible. Running is your first line of defense. If running isn't an option, then you do what you have to do to protect your family. Fighting back should always be on the table, but only as a last resort. Your job is to make sure that things never get that far.

LET YOUR FAMILY GET IN THE CAR FIRST

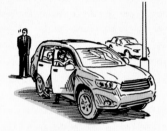

STAND AT the back of the car while your family gets in. If you're in the car before your family gets in and an attack does happen, you're at a tactical disadvantage. Threats aren't always attackers. It could be a little old lady who's backing up her boat of a Cadillac and can't see that she's about to hit your kid.

Take precautions, but try not to look like a weirdo while doing so.

WHEN STOPPED IN YOUR VEHICLE, BE SURE YOU CAN SEE THE TIRES OF THE CAR IN FRONT OF YOU

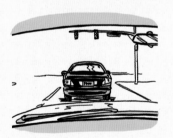

WHILE YOU'LL likely never have to utilize a Rockford J-Turn to escape from bad guys, make sure you can see the tires of the car in front of you when stopped at an intersection.

MAKE A PERFECT OMELET

The omelet is the star among all egg-centric breakfast dishes. It can be as simple as plain or featuring just ham and cheddar; or you can branch out and add various meats, cheeses, and vegetables. It makes for a great dish for both the bachelor looking for a quick and healthy breakfast (or breakfast for dinner), or the dad making Saturday morning goodness for his family.

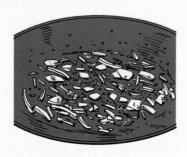

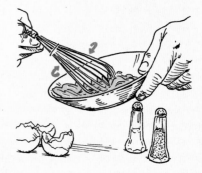

1: PREHEAT a medium-size skillet on medium-high. Sauté the fillings—veggies, ham, etc.—3–4 minutes, until tender.

2: MEANWHILE, whisk 3 eggs until frothy, seasoning liberally with salt and pepper.

The key to the perfect omelet is a little finesse.

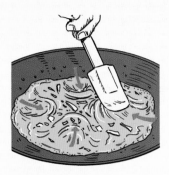

3: ADD eggs to skillet, with veggies, and let cook undisturbed for a minute. Next, gently pull the eggs from the outside to the center, allowing the liquid to flow underneath and cook.

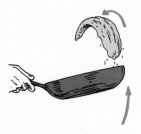

4: WHEN eggs are mostly set, flip. Do this with a spatula, or for the seasoned chef, use the edge of the skillet and some upward force.

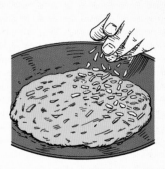

5: SPRINKLE cheese on one side; cook for an additional minute.

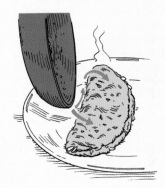

6: SERVE omelet out of the skillet by folding it in half as you set it on the plate. Allow cheese to melt for 30 seconds, and enjoy!

BE AN AWESOME UNCLE

Uncles exist in a magical world. Old enough to look after their nieces and nephews, but not so old as to be out of touch, uncles offer advice without seeming overbearing and fun experiences without seeming lame. Navigating that balance as a cool advisor isn't without its challenges.

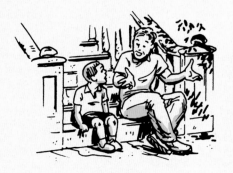

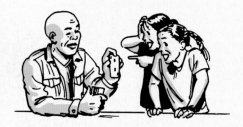

1: OFFER advice when appropriate. Let them know you're available if they have questions or need to talk to someone.

2: UNCLES are the epitome of fun and cool, so bone up on jokes, riddles, and magic tricks.

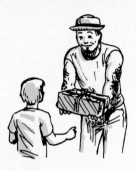

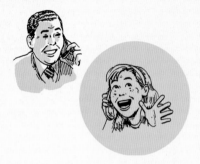

3: GET them cool gifts on their birthdays and holidays. Can't think of anything? A pile of green will always work!

5: BE a consistent fixture in their life by attending sporting events, making regular phone calls, and visiting them.

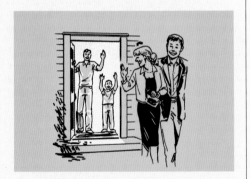

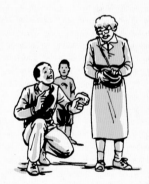

4: OFFER to babysit. It offers support to your siblings and it allows you to spend meaningful one-on-one time with your niece or nephew.

6: ACT as an example by being a gentleman in every interaction, not just with your niece or nephew.

COOL UNCLE TRICKS

An essential part of being an awesome uncle is developing a repertoire of tricks and jokes that will amaze your nieces and nephews, and crack them up.

HOW TO LEVITATE

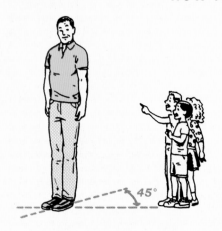

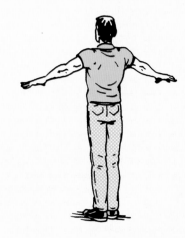

1: STAND in front of your audience, facing away from them, with your body positioned at about a 45-degree angle from them. You want them to be able to only see your left foot and heel, and the back of your right heel.

2: DRAMATICALLY lift arms with your palms facing down so as to give the impression you're about to push down and lift yourself off the ground.

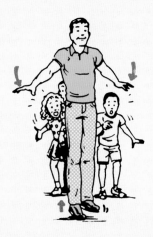

3: PUSH down with your hands, while simultaneously lifting yourself up on your right hidden toes. Keep both heels together as your feet rise.

*All kids love to play;
play along with them.*

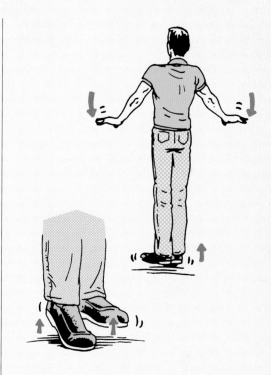

4: HOLD for two to three seconds and then let yourself down. Lower yourself slowly, or drop dramatically as if you've sapped yourself of all magical energy.

HOW TO BOUNCE A ROLL

A GREAT mealtime gag: "bouncing" a dinner roll on the floor. You can also bounce a donut at breakfast, or any other suitable baked good. The trick works best when you're sitting at a table with a tablecloth that will hide what's really going on. But you can do it at any table, as long as you keep your audience's eyes above the tabletop.

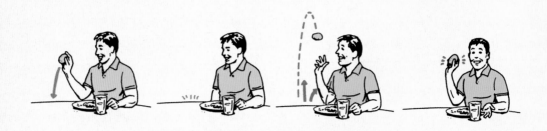

What It Looks Like

1: YOU are seen throwing the roll on the floor.

2: THE sound of the roll hitting the floor is heard.

3: THE roll pops up.

4: YOU catch the roll triumphantly.

An uncle is there to help a child get into mischief they haven't thought of yet.

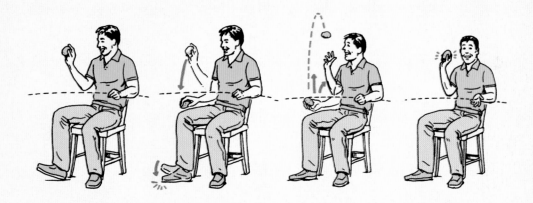

What's Actually Happening

1: FOOT is ready to stamp.

2: TAP your foot on the ground to make the "bouncing" sound.

3: TOSS the roll back up into the air.

4: CATCH the roll. Await applause from nieces and nephews.

HOW TO MAKE A GRASS WHISTLE

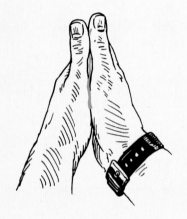

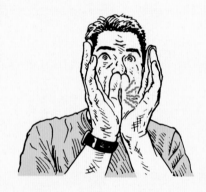

1: PLACE a nice thick blade of grass between your two thumbs.

2: PLACE back of thumbs against your mouth and blow! You know you're successful by the annoying screeching sound coming out from your thumbs.

The best cool uncle tricks entertain the kids—and annoy the adults.

THE WORLD'S GREATEST PAPER AIRPLANE

From the earliest paper planes developed in China 2,000 years ago through the parchment planes Leonardo da Vinci made to test his aerial designs, the paper airplane has fascinated generations. New styles that soar hundreds of feet and stay in the air for nearly half a minute are being dreamed up by ingenious folders around the world. But we like this paper airplane, called the Harrier, the best. It is the perfect middle ground between simplicity and performance.

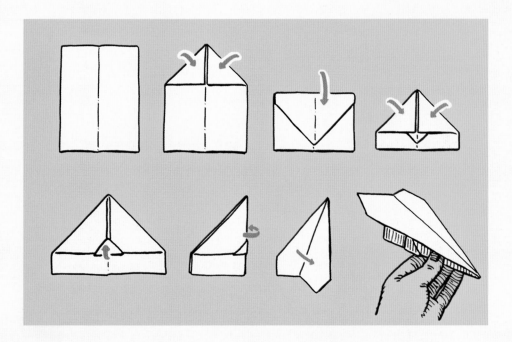

SKIP A STONE

Skipping a stone on water is a fun way to while away the time on a camping trip or picnic—exactly the kind of analog distraction that helps you navigate your thoughts if you're alone, or lets a deep conversation with a friend run its course. Centuries of fathers and sons have discussed the meaning of life standing by the edge of a pond, stones in hand. This is something you'll want to pass on to your kids.

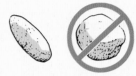

1: PICK the right stone: flat, uniform thickness/thinness, fits in your palm, and no heavier than a tennis ball. Too heavy and the rock won't skip off the water.

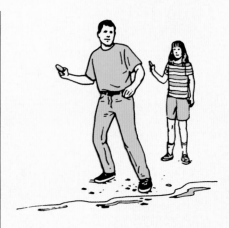

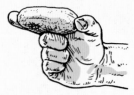

2: HOLD the stone between your thumb and middle finger, with your thumb on top, and your index finger hooked along the edge.

3: STAND facing the water at a slight angle. With rock in hand, pull your arm back like you're going to throw a sidearm pitch.

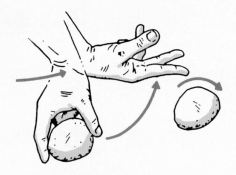

4: AS you throw the rock, cock your wrist back. Right before the release, give your wrist a quick flick. This will create the spin needed for the stone to skip across the water.

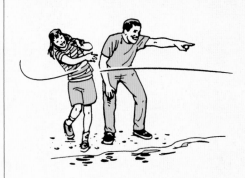

6: HAVE fun skipping stones with your kiddos!

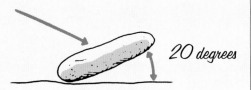

20 degrees

5: THROW out and down at the same time. For maximum skips, the stone should enter the water at a 20-degree angle. Scientists have found this to be the optimal angle!

What we plant in the soil of contemplation, we shall reap in the harvest of action.

— Meister Eckhart

Chapter 6

The
LEADER

Leadership is the art of getting someone else to do something you want done because he wants to do it.

—Dwight D. Eisenhower

THROUGHOUT HISTORY, the right leader has often appeared at exactly the right time. Washington during the Revolution. Lincoln during the Civil War. Churchill during the Big One. We recall these great leaders as though they were destined to rise to the occasion. But look closely at their careers, and you'll see they developed their leadership skills with great discipline and dedication.

Long before he became the masterful general and statesman we now know, Washington suffered devastating setbacks in battle at the beginning of the War of Independence. Lincoln failed in business and in several political campaigns before he became the Great Emancipator. And as the First Lord of the Admiralty during World War I, Churchill made a disastrous strategic decision that resulted in his being dismissed and excluded from the War Council. Twenty-five years later, he led Great Britain in their "finest hour."

LEADERS AREN'T BORN. THEY'RE MADE — OFTEN IN THE FURNACE OF SETBACKS.

We may not be called upon to lead men into battle or a guide a country through its darkest time, but the attributes of the finest leaders in history are the same ones we must cultivate to lead our families, businesses, and communities to higher ground.

THE FIVE TRAITS OF LEADERSHIP

Shortly after World War II, the US military published a booklet outlining five key leadership traits every soldier should develop. These traits are just as applicable to civilians who strive to be better leaders in their everyday lives. Taken together, they can help define, create, and support leaders in all positions.

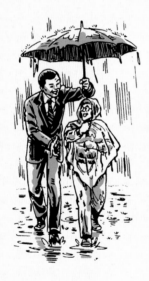

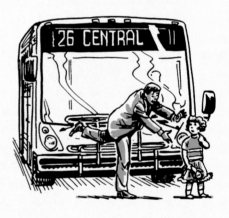

1: EXEMPLIFY quiet resolution by sticking to your values, committing to your decisions, and standing strong throughout crises when they develop.

2: BE willing to take risks when necessary.

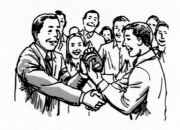

3: REWARD subordinates when their efforts have helped your team succeed.

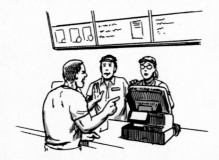

4: TAKE your equal share of blame when things go wrong.

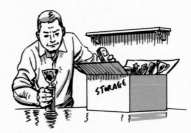

5: DO not dwell on past successes or failures. Rather, focus on future goals.

THE EISENHOWER DECISION MATRIX

A leader makes decisions. But with a flood of tasks coming your way, you can spend more time managing crises and putting out fires than making meaningful progress. If you find yourself constantly treading water, you have likely confused urgency with importance.

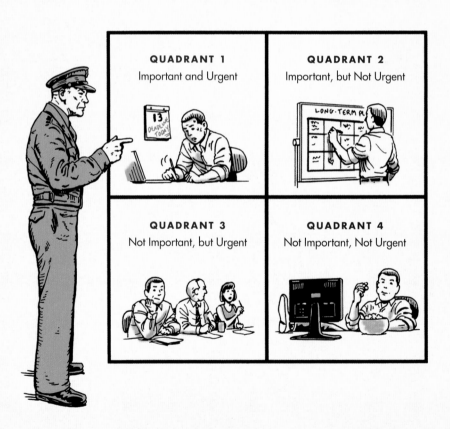

DWIGHT D. Eisenhower knew a lot about making tough decisions. As the Supreme Commander of the largest amphibious military invasion in human history and later as President of the United States, Eisenhower had to make a lot of them. He was able to remain effective by reminding himself of this principle: "What is important is seldom urgent and what is urgent is seldom important."

EFFECTIVE LEADERS spend more time on the important tasks and less time on the urgent ones. The hard part is figuring out which is which. To give you a jump start, we present the Eisenhower Decision Matrix. Spend as much time as possible in Quadrant 2, and you'll be the Supreme Commander of your day.

"What is important is seldom urgent and what is urgent is seldom important."

—Dwight D. Eisenhower

THE OODA LOOP

John Boyd is perhaps the greatest unknown military strategist in history. His most significant contribution is an incredible strategic tool: the OODA Loop — Observe, Orient, Decide, Act. It models the process that human beings and organizations use to learn, grow, and thrive in rapidly changing environments—in war, business, and life.

THE OODA Loop is sometimes misdescribed as a four-step process where the one who makes it through all the stages the quickest wins. There's more to it than that. For the full range of nuance, pick up *Science, Strategy and War* by Frans P. B. Osinga.

THE OODA Loop is based on the belief that we are hindered by an inability to rapidly make sense of a changing reality. When circumstances change, we fail to revise our mental models and struggle to see the world as we feel it should be, rather than how it really is.

This is the loop's most basic version:

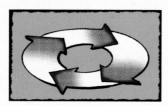

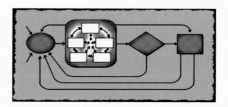

1: BOYD himself used this diagram when explaining the Loop, but his full vision was grander:

2: THE full Loop can look like gobbledy-gook to the uninitiated. But once you understand the thinking behind this diagram, you'll realize how profound it is.

OBSERVE

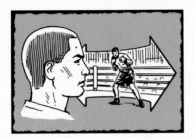

TAKING IN new information about our environment is crucial in revising the mental models we use to make decisions. But we often observe imperfect or incomplete information, and we can be inundated with so much of it that we can't separate the signal from the noise. We address this uncertainty by developing our judgment—by orienting ourselves.

ORIENT

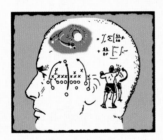

OUR ORIENTATION shapes how we observe, decide, and act. To orient yourself in a changing environment, you must constantly break apart old mental models and reassemble them to better match reality. This is a continual process: As soon as you create a new mental concept, it becomes outdated as the environment around you changes. Boyd offered this advice on orientation:

Build a robust toolbox of mental models.

BOYD LAYS out seven disciplines you ought to know: Mathematical Logic, Physics, Thermodynamics, Biology, Psychology, Anthropology, and Conflict (Game Theory). To thrive in your job, you also need mental models specific to your career. To survive a lethal encounter, you'll need models unique to tactical situations. Learn as many models as you can.

Start destroying and creating mental models.

WHEN YOU'RE faced with a new problem, go through the domains above and ask, "Are there elements from these different mental concepts that can provide insight into my problem?"

Never stop orienting.

BECAUSE THE world around you is constantly changing, orientation is something you can never stop doing. "Always Be Orienting" should become your mantra. Make it a goal to add to your mental toolbox every day.

Try to validate mental models before operation.

STUDY WHAT mental concepts have and haven't worked in similar situations and then practice, train, and visualize using those mental concepts.

DECIDE (HYPOTHESIS)

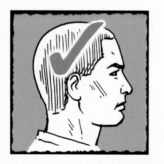

IT'S IMPOSSIBLE to select a perfect mental model because of the uncertainty inherent in a changing world. Consequently, when we pair a mental model with the information we have, we're forced to settle for ones that we guess are good enough. To find out if our hypothesis is correct, we then have to test it.

ACT (TEST)

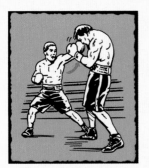

THE OODA Loop is not only a decision process, but a learning system. By constantly "experimenting" we improve how we operate in every facet of our lives. Action is how we find out if our mental models are correct. If they are, we win the battle; if they aren't, then we start the OODA Loop again using newly observed data.

TEMPO

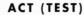

To the Swift Goes the Race

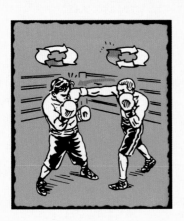

THE OODA Loop can guide our individual actions and doesn't require an "opponent" per se in order to be useful. But in situations of conflict or competition, where it's your OODA Loop going head-to-head against someone else's, tempo is important.

THOSE WHO cycle through successful, consecutive OODA Loops faster than their opponents will win in a conflict. Rapid OODA Looping on your part "resets" your opponent's OODA Loop by causing confusion—it sends them back to the observation phase to figure out how to proceed. The key to speed is practice.

DEVELOP CHARISMA

Charisma is what allows you to command a room, draws others to you, and convinces people of your success. It's an essential part of being a leader. Charismatic men are perceived as both likable and powerful: a dynamic, irresistible combination that can open endless doors.

Far from a magical or inexplicable trait, charisma comes from a set of concrete, largely nonverbal behaviors that can be learned. Olivia Fox Cabane, author of *The Charisma Myth*, places the behaviors that produce strong personal magnetism into three categories: Presence, Power, and Warmth.

PRESENCE

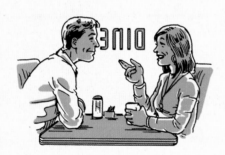

1: THE paradox of charisma is that it's not about trumpeting your good qualities, but making the other person feel good about him- or herself. Real charisma makes the other person feel important—that you were actually present with them.

2: BRING yourself to the here and now. If your mind is somewhere else, focus for a second or two on physical sensations that you often ignore: your breath or your feet touching the ground.

3: LOOK the person in the eye when they're talking. Eye contact imparts a sense of intimacy to your exchanges, and leaves the receiver of your gaze feeling more connected to you.

4: ASK clarifying questions. Show that you're completely there by asking questions after he or she has spoken. Paraphrase what the person said and add, "Am I understanding you correctly?"

5: WAIT before responding. Breaking in the instant a person pauses sends the signal that you were only thinking about what you wanted to say instead of listening to them. Waiting two seconds before you respond will convey that you've taken in what they said.

POWER

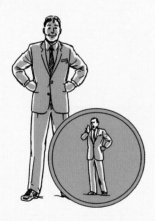

1: OFFERING a first impression of power mainly comes down to enhancing the things humans are wired to register: body language and appearance.

2: BECOME physically fit. A fit, muscular physique sends a signal to the most primal parts of other people's brains about your strength and ability to dominate and protect.

3: DRESS for power. Instead of a t-shirt, don a nice button-down shirt, a pair of khakis, and some leather dress boots. Slip on a sport coat or blazer to create a more masculine silhouette.

4: TAKE up space. Look for ways to subtly increase the amount of space you take up when seated, and assume power poses (like with your arms akimbo, hands resting on the waist) when standing.

5: SPEAK less and more slowly. Powerful people take up space in conversation—but don't hog the speaking time. They speak less and aren't afraid of "awkward" silence. People often nervously try to fill silent gaps, which is why interrogators and negotiators resort to the silent treatment.

6: KNOW a little about a lot. Intelligence is a key marker of a man who is able to affect the world around him. Read every chance you get. Seek to know as much about as many subjects as possible in addition to one area of expertise.

WARMTH

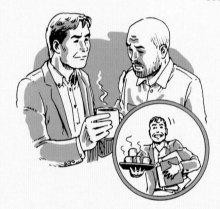

1: WHEN you emanate Warmth people feel at ease. Warmth fulfills the basic human need to be understood, acknowledged, and cared for. Of all the elements of charisma, warmth is the hardest to fake. People are

pretty good at sniffing out fake warmth, and tend to recoil when they're offered the counterfeit variety. The behaviors that communicate warmth to others arise from that most powerful but ineffable quality: a genuinely good heart. You can develop your inner warmth by practicing gratitude empathy on a daily basis, and it's well worth the effort.

2: THINK of yourself as the host. When you have people over to your house, you look for ways to make them feel comfortable. Bring this same mentality to all your interactions.

3: SMILE when you speak. This puts more warmth in your voice, and is especially useful when talking on the phone.

4: MIRROR their body language. When you mirror a person's body language and manner of speaking, they'll trust you and find you more attractive. Don't match your conversation partner tic for tic, but if they speak softly, bring your own voice down a notch; if they lean back in their chair, lean back just a bit, too. Let a few seconds lapse before you move into a mirrored position.

5: RELAX your posture and open up. While an erect posture creates the perception of power and confidence, it can sometimes make you seem stiff or haughty. Instead of crossing your arms, keep them by your side; instead of crossing your legs, leave them open. Remove barriers between you and the other person.

6: SMILE, dammit! It makes you more attractive and approachable.

7: REMEMBER dates, anniversaries, and details. It's amazing how far remembering someone's birthday will go with people. Send a card or an email—take the chance not only to wish them happy birthday but to say hello and ask how they are.

8: BE liberal with the thank you notes. They tell people you noticed and took the time to acknowledge them. It's warmth in an envelope.

Charismatic men are perceived as both likable and powerful: a dynamic, irresistible combination that can open endless doors.

ACHIEVE MANLY POSTURE

When we sit or stand with good posture we improve our breathing, memory, and learning ability. It delivers confidence and a powerful presence. Good posture can even make you feel manly by boosting your testosterone.

GOOD POSTURE should not feel rigid or take a lot of work. With good posture, your bones, not your muscles, keep your body upright and balanced. Your overall goal is to have a "neutral spine" that retains three natural curves: a small hollow at the neck's base, a small roundness at the middle back, and a small hollow in the lower back.

STANDING

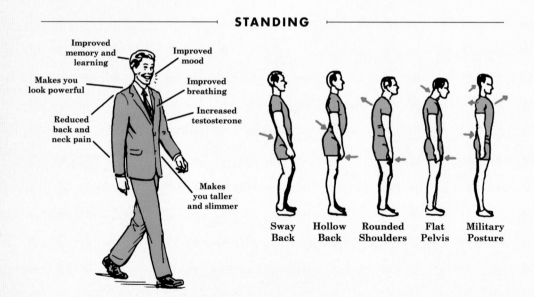

Improved memory and learning

Improved mood

Makes you look powerful

Improved breathing

Increased testosterone

Reduced back and neck pain

Makes you taller and slimmer

Sway Back · Hollow Back · Rounded Shoulders · Flat Pelvis · Military Posture

IMAGINE A plumb line running from your earlobe. With correct posture, the line hangs straight to the middle of your anklebone, with your shoulders, hips, and knees in a straight line. If you have a hard time making your body fit that mental picture, do this wall exercise:

STAND WITH head, shoulders, and back against a wall and your heels 5–6 inches forward. Draw in the lower abdominal muscles, decreasing the arch in your lower back. This is what good posture feels like. Now push away from the wall and maintain this upright, vertical alignment.

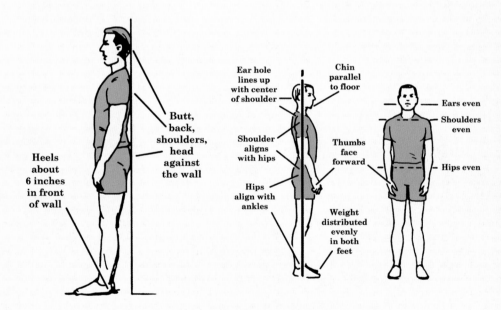

Heels about 6 inches in front of wall

Butt, back, shoulders, head against the wall

Ear hole lines up with center of shoulder

Chin parallel to floor

Shoulder aligns with hips

Thumbs face forward

Hips align with ankles

Weight distributed evenly in both feet

Ears even

Shoulders even

Hips even

SITTING

Poor Posture When Sitting

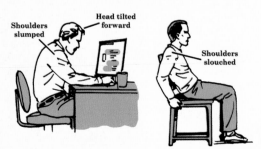

Shoulders slumped

Head tilted forward

Shoulders slouched

Good Posture When Sitting

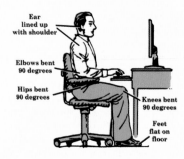

Ear lined up with shoulder

Elbows bent 90 degrees

Hips bent 90 degrees

Knees bent 90 degrees

Feet flat on floor

IT'S HARDER to maintain good posture while sitting than standing, so the first thing you can do is start sitting less. Take a break every thirty to forty-five minutes to get up and move. Consider using a standing desk in moderation, alternating between sitting and standing throughout the day.

WHEN YOU do sit, keep your ears and shoulders lined up but relaxed, and make sure your feet rest flat on the floor, with your knees and hips bent 90 degrees. Your elbows should also bend at 90 degrees while typing. If your knees, hips, and elbows aren't bent correctly, adjust your chair until they are.

AVOID THE SMARTPHONE SLUMP

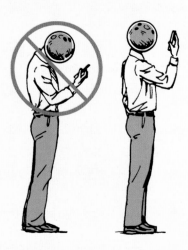

WHEN YOU have good posture, your head lines up on top of your spinal column. The force you exert to keep your head in this neutral position is equal to the weight of your head—about eleven pounds. But as you move your head forward, the force needed to keep your head up increases. When you tilt your head forward 45 degrees, it's exerting almost fifty pounds of force on your neck.

SMARTPHONE SLUMP wreaks havoc on your muscles and may even factor into the rise of depression in the West. (A slouched, submissive position can lead to low mood.) But fixing Smartphone Slump is easy: Don't look down at your phone. Instead, bring your phone up to eye level. Yes, you'll look like you're constantly taking selfies, but it will keep that big ol' bowling ball of a head balanced on top of your spine—and relieve the muscles in your back, shoulders, and neck.

A slouched posture can lead to low mood.

DE-QUASIMODO YOURSELF

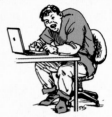

Poor sitting posture can cause jaw aches and headaches, and in the long term it can result in kyphosis, or a permanently visible hump on your upper back. Kyphosis isn't just an aesthetic problem—it can cause pain and breathing difficulties. Here are six exercises to counteract the ill effects of slouching. Consider it your de-Quasimodo routine.

Doorway Stretch

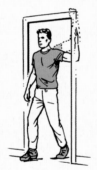

1: STAND inside a doorway (or next to a squat rack at the gym). Bend your right arm 90 degrees (like you're giving a high five) and place your forearm against the door frame. Position your bent elbow at about shoulder height. Rotate your chest left until you feel a nice stretch in your chest and front shoulder. Hold it for thirty seconds. Repeat with the opposite arm.

2: STRETCH different parts of your chest by moving your elbow on the door frame.

The lower your elbow, the more your pectoralis major gets stretched; the higher your elbow, the more you stretch your pectoralis minor.

Pectoral Ball Smash

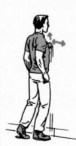

1: LOOSEN up tight muscles in your chest by doing some trigger point release with a lacrosse ball.

2: PLACE the ball between your chest and the wall. Roll the ball around on your chest until you find a "hot spot"—you know you've found one if it hurts when the ball rolls over it. When you find a trigger point, stop and just rest on the ball for ten to twenty seconds. It's this pressure, not the rolling, that smoothes fascia and releases tight, knotty muscles. Continue rolling and finding more trigger spots. Do a five-minute session three times a week.

Shoulder Dislocations

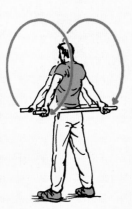

1: DON'T worry, you don't actually dislocate your shoulders with this exercise! But this movement does wonders for loosening up shoulders that have become tight from years of turning inward while slouching.

2: YOU'LL need a PVC pipe or broomstick that's about five feet in length. Hold the PVC pipe in front of you with an overhand grip. If your shoulders are really inflexible, start off with a pretty wide grip—as wide as possible. As your flexibility increases, narrow your grip.

3: SLOWLY lift the PVC pipe in front of you, then over your head, until it hits you in the back/butt area. Then come back to the starting position. Again, do this SLOWLY. If you do it too fast, you're likely to injure yourself. Do three sets of 10 reps.

Thoracic Extension on Foam Roller

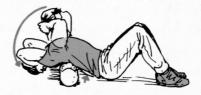

1: PLACE the foam roller under your upper back. Your feet and butt should be on the floor. Place your hands behind your head and bring your elbows as close together as you can. Let your head drop to the floor, and try to "wrap" yourself around the foam roller. Begin to roll the foam roller up and down your back, searching for "hot spots." When you find one, lift your head up and really dig your back into the foam roller. Lay your head back down and continue searching for more hot spots along your thoracic spine (the middle of your back).

Prone Y Extension

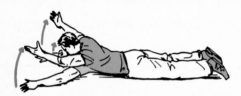

1: LIE facedown on the floor and put your hands above your head in a "Y" position with your palms facing down. Lift up your torso, just as you would with a back extension, while externally rotating your shoulders so that your palms face each other at the top of the movement. Keep your head in line with your neck and back. Hold that position for five to ten seconds. Lower yourself down to the starting position and repeat ten more times.

Wall Angels

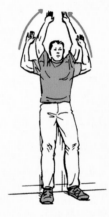

1: IT may not look like it, but this exercise will have you grunting in pain after a few reps.

2: START with knees slightly bent, and your lower back, upper back, and head pressed against the wall. Arms are also on the wall, with your fingers pushed against it. Think of giving the "It's good!" football sign.

3: MOVE your arms up above your head, like a snow angel. The key is to keep your fingers, entire back and butt, and head pushing into the wall. The tendency will be to arch out. If your backside loses contact with the wall, you're doing it wrong.

BECOME A T-SHAPED MAN

You've probably desired a V-shaped physical body, but there's an ideal shape for your mental "physique" too: the T. A T-shaped man has expertise in one skill or discipline, as well as a broader range of skills and knowledge. He is a jack-of-all-trades, and a master of one.

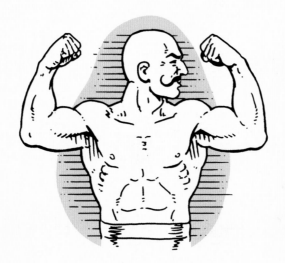

Many of history's most eminent men were T-shaped. Think of Leonardo da Vinci: a master artist who also studied and dabbled in anatomy, mechanics, architecture, and botany. Instead of diluting his artistic ability, his broad interests made him a better artist. His study of human anatomy enabled him to paint and sculpt the most lifelike depictions of the human form up to that point in history. His interest in mechanics led him to sketch concepts that were hundreds of years ahead of their time, like tanks, helicopters, and airplanes. Follow his example by gaining mastery in one domain while dabbling in several others.

UNDO THE DAMAGE OF SITTING

Besides causing a Quasimodo hunch, sitting for long periods of time can cause lots of tightness in your hips. But loose hips are an essential part of a healthy and robust body. First, having limber hips just feels good, plain and simple. Second, having a healthy range of motion in your hips can help prevent injury when you pursue more recreational physical activities and do household chores. For example, loose hips keep your IT band loose as well, which can ward off knee pain. Finally, taking care of your hips may help improve your posture, which can in turn alleviate back or neck pain. (Not to mention the role of limber hips in doing a mean mambo.)

Below, we provide some simple stretches and exercises that will undo the damage to your hips caused by sitting at a desk all day.

PREVENTION IS THE BEST REMEDY: SIT LESS AND MOVE MORE

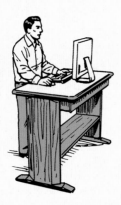

AS THE saying goes, "an ounce of prevention is worth a pound of cure." The best thing you can do for your hip mobility is to simply sit less and move more during the day.

IF YOUR employer will allow it, try using a standing desk, which keeps your muscles activated at the office. Keep in mind that, just as with sitting, standing should be done in moderation (doing it for an extended period of time isn't that great for you, either). If a standing desk isn't an option, take five-minute breaks from sitting every thirty to forty-five minutes. Stand up and walk around a bit. Maybe even perform a few of the exercises below. Even if you have a standing desk, you should still take breaks every now and then for some movement.

STRETCH OUT THOSE HIPS

IF YOU'RE really tight, take it nice and easy with these exercises. As physical therapist Kelly Starrett says, "Don't go into the pain cave. Your animal totem won't be there to help you."

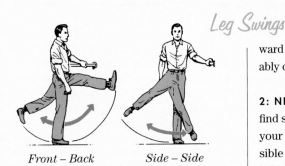

Front – Back   *Side – Side*

1: BEGIN with forward leg swings. Find something to hold for balance. Start off swinging your right leg backward and for-ward as high and as far back as you comfortably can. Do 20 swings and then switch legs.

2: NEXT are side-to-side swings. Again, find something to hold for balance. Swing your right leg out to the side as high as possible and then in front of you toward your left as far as you can go. Perform 20 swings and then switch legs. Depending on how tight you feel, you may need another set.

Grok Squat

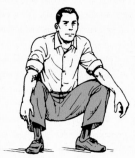

THE GROK Squat is similar to a catcher's stance in baseball. Simply squat down until your butt touches your ankles. Keep your heels firmly on the ground and your back straight. Hold that position for thirty to sixty seconds. You should feel your hamstrings, quads, Achilles tendons, lower back, and groin gently stretching. If you're super stiff, it may take a few days of practice to sink into a full squat. Keep at it. Your back and hips will thank you. Intersperse a few short squatting sessions into your daily routine.

Table Pigeon Pose

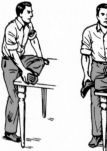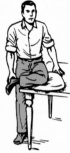

Harder   *Easier*

IF YOU'VE done yoga, you're probably familiar with the pigeon pose. This stretch is the same thing, except you use a table, which makes it a bit easier to perform and allows you to stretch out your muscles from different angles. Start by placing your leg on a tabletop (you could also use your bed) with the knee bent at 90 degrees. Place one hand on the table and one hand on your foot for support. Lean forward and hold for sixty to ninety seconds. Then lean left to the ten o'clock position and hold for sixty to ninety seconds. Lean right to the two o'clock position and hold for sixty to ninety seconds. Repeat on the other leg.

IF YOU have knee problems, rotate your body so that your ankle hangs off the table and place a pillow underneath your knee. Aim to do two pigeon poses a day (I personally do one during my workout and another at a random time).

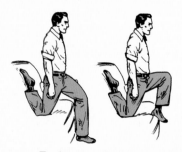

Easier   *Harder*

Couch Stretch

THE COUCH stretch is basically a quad stretch ratcheted up a few notches. It will undo years of sitting. You actually don't need a couch for this stretch, it just makes it a bit more comfortable (if that's even possible). You can also do it on the floor by putting your knee against a wall.

FOR THE "easy" version, place the knee of the leg you're stretching against the back of your sofa. Place the foot of your other leg on the floor. Slowly raise your torso to a neutral spine position (i.e., standing straight and tall). As you raise your torso, squeeze your butt and abs. Hold the position for up to four minutes. Switch and repeat on the other leg. You should feel things really stretch in your hip flexor area—just don't push yourself too hard.

TO UP the ante, bring your non-stretching leg up onto the seat of the couch. Keeping a straight, neutral spine, squeeze the butt and abs and work your way up to holding the position for four minutes. Keep in mind that it may be awhile before you can get your torso to a straight position. When I first started doing this stretch the "hard way," I could only raise my torso to a 45-degree angle and I'd have to support myself with my hand on the floor. I was eventually able to move to a straight position after two weeks of dedicated stretching. The difference in the mobility of my hips was (and continues to be) significant.

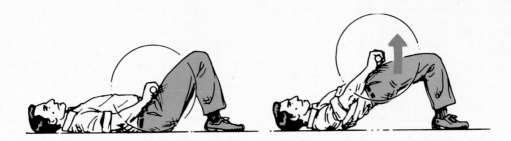

Barbell Glute Bridge

ENTER AND EXIT A ROOM LIKE A MAN

When you meet someone for the first time, put your best foot forward. That starts with how you enter a room—and how you leave. Make a good impression and you'll kickstart a positive relationship.

ENTRY

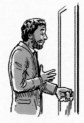

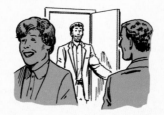

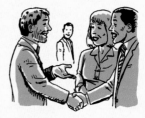

1: HAVE a firm sense of purpose as you step through the door. Don't enter until you're ready.

2: ENTER with a smile and good posture. Straighten your back and raise your head so that you're looking across the room, not at the floor.

3: GREET people warmly, gesticulating as you speak with articulation.

No matter how smoothly you do it, a graceful exit is impossible if it's at the wrong time.

EXIT

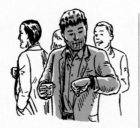 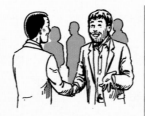 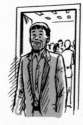

1: DECIDE when it's appropriate to leave. For a stop-in party, wait at least an hour to leave. For dinner, wait until after dessert or coffee is served.

2: STAND up, shake hands with the host, gather your things, say "thank you," and offer your good-byes.

3: COMMIT to leaving as you walk to the door and make your exit. Don't get caught talking to someone on your way out, it only invalidates your need to leave.

END A CONVERSATION

We've all ended up in conversations that have gone on too long. But leaving a conversation abruptly can leave the other person feeling rejected, unless you do it with grace. And you can! Stop that unfortunate chitchat in its tracks by making sure you have a clear reason to leave the conversation in mind, waiting for a lull to make your move, and then executing your break with purpose.

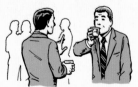

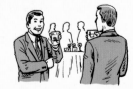

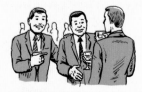

1: WAIT for a lull in the conversation, like a long pause between sentences or when the other person takes a drink. That's your time to act.

2: USE an exit line. Tell the person you have to ask someone a question, get a drink, or check on something.

3: INTRODUCE the person to someone else at the party, or ask to be introduced to someone the person knows.

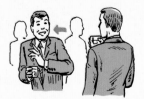

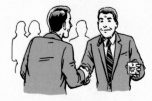

4: INVITE the person to do something with you. The change of scenery may prompt the conversation to end.

5: LET them know it was nice to speak with them, shake their hand, and exit with purpose. If you used an exit line, make sure to follow through with the excuse you used.

DRESS FOR A JOB INTERVIEW

You want to put your best foot forward during a job interview, and your appearance is a big part of that. You want to look presentable, well-groomed, and dressed appropriately for the type of job you're applying for. A good general rule to follow is to dress one notch up from that workplace's dress code. If you're applying to a restaurant where the waiters wear jeans and t-shirts, wear khakis and a polo shirt to the interview. If you're applying to a place where people wear khakis and polos, then wear a button-down shirt and khakis to the interview. If everyone wears khakis and button-down shirts, then do likewise, but add a sport coat and tie. You get the idea.

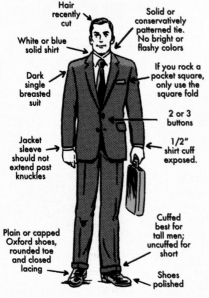

Hair recently cut

White or blue solid shirt

Dark single breasted suit

Jacket sleeve should not extend past knuckles

Solid or conservatively patterned tie. No bright or flashy colors

If you rock a pocket square, only use the square fold

2 or 3 buttons

1/2" shirt cuff exposed.

Plain or capped Oxford shoes, rounded toe and closed lacing

Cuffed best for tall men; uncuffed for short

Shoes polished

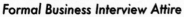

Formal Business Interview Attire

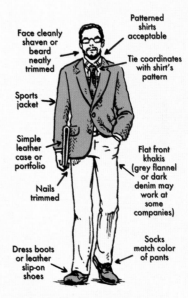

Face cleanly shaven or beard neatly trimmed

Sports jacket

Simple leather case or portfolio

Nails trimmed

Dress boots or leather slip-on shoes

Patterned shirts acceptable

Tie coordinates with shirt's pattern

Flat front khakis (grey flannel or dark denim may work at some companies)

Socks match color of pants

Casual Job Interview Attire

THINGS EVERY MAN
SHOULD HAVE IN HIS DESK

An office desk is your home away from home. It keeps you organized and comfortable, whether you're a graphic designer in a skyscraper or a middle school teacher in a rural Midwest town. Stock it with essential items and a few emergency supplies.

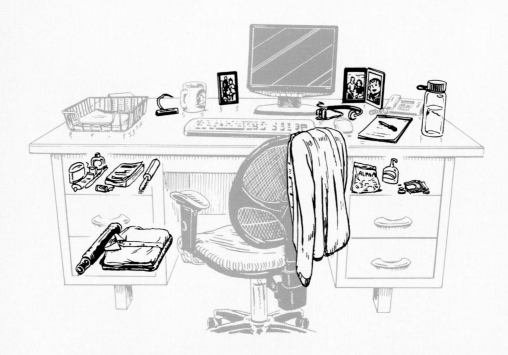

With these essentials, you're prepared for any workplace event—or accident.

1: CLOTHES—A spare suit jacket for impromptu but important meetings, a sweater to manage aggressive A/C, and a spare shirt and pants in the event of a spill.

2: TOILETRIES—Deodorant, a toothbrush and toothpaste, floss, and cologne.

3: LINT ROLLER

4: BREATH MINTS

5: HAND SANITIZER

6: SNACKS—Something healthy with a long shelf life, like almonds.

7: FRAMED PICTURES—Of family and friends.

8: CASH—$20 in bills and coins should do it.

9: NOVEL—To read over lunch and to rest your eyes from heavy screen usage for five to ten minutes every hour.

10: HEADPHONES—A godsend for your produc-tivity, especially in cubicle farms.

11: WATER BOTTLE—Stay hydrated and eliminate waste.

12: PHONE CHARGER

13: UMBRELLA

14: NOTEBOOK AND PEN

RUN A MEETING

From intense corporate gatherings at the top of gleaming skyscrapers to the team get-togethers at mom and pop restaurants, work meetings are an essential part of getting key staff members to talk about issues important to the business. As important as they can be, though, too many meetings are a waste of time. Distracted participants, tangential topics, and a lack of focus can result in a lack of productivity and few concrete benefits. When you're in charge of a meeting, rise to the challenge with specific ideas and an action plan to get things done.

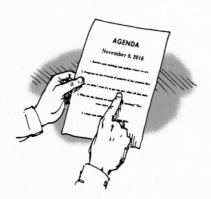

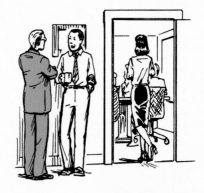

1: **TYPE** up an agenda for the meeting with a specific list of what items will be discussed and in what order.

2: **MAKE** sure key people will be in attendance, and resolve any pet issues one on one before the meeting.

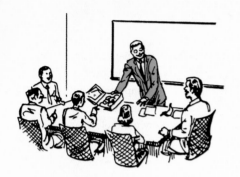

3: BRING bagels or donuts, set up the chairs in a U-shape, and start on time.

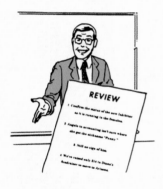

4: BEGIN with what was accomplished since the last meeting.

5: GET to the heart of the meeting, come up with tangible solutions to problems, and control the discussion to stay on track.

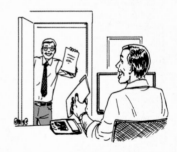

6: SUMMARIZE the meeting, end on time, and follow-up to make sure things get done.

MAKE A PITCH

Whether you're a writer trying to sell your book idea to a publisher, a sous chef trying to convince your boss to put your dish on the menu, or a husband who wants to move his family to Florida so he can pursue his dream of becoming an astronaut, a pitch is the way to convince someone that they need to act on your idea.

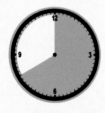

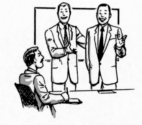

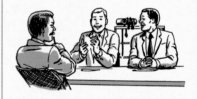

1: SCHEDULE a meeting for earlier in the day, when people have more energy.

2: HAVE a partner help you make the pitch, establishing each person's role before you do it.

3: DELIVER the pitch with a casual tone, avoiding PowerPoints, and starting a conversation that finds common ground with the buyer.

Stay cool and collected under pressure.

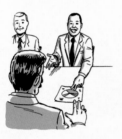

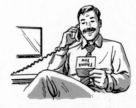

4: BEGIN with the most important details that get to the core of your idea, emphasizing why your idea is so great, and tie in reasons why your buyer is perfectly suited for your idea.

5: ANTICIPATE concerns and have answers prepared for their possible questions in advance.

6: CLOSE with a clear request, ask how you can resolve their issues if they say "no," and always follow-up after the meeting with a phone call and a note, regardless of their answer.

BASICS OF OFFICE ETIQUETTE

The modern office environment is a world away from what it was a few decades ago. Collaborative work spaces, dog-friendly offices, and recreation rooms with everything from ping pong tables to bean bags have replaced the formal workspaces where we used to clock in and out. But, even with a more casual trend in the working world, there are still rules for behaving in a way that respects your coworkers and the environment where you and your officemates take care of business.

DO

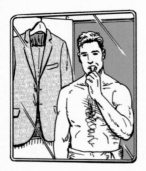 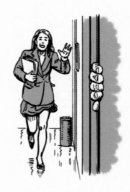 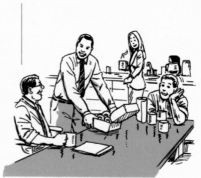

1: DRESS with respect and maintain a high level of hygiene.

2: HOLD the door for people trying to get on the elevator.

3: BRING snacks or treats to share with coworkers every once in a while.

The modern office environment is a world away from what it was a few decades ago.

DON'T

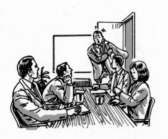

1: COME late to meetings.

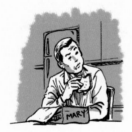

2: EAT other people's food out of communal kitchens.

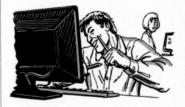

3: LISTEN to music or videos without headphones.

GIVE A MANLY HANDSHAKE

Whether greeting someone for the first or the hundredth time, a good handshake conveys confidence, strength, warmth, honesty, and a host of other character traits. A confident, successful handshake boils down to three keys: how, when, and where you do it.

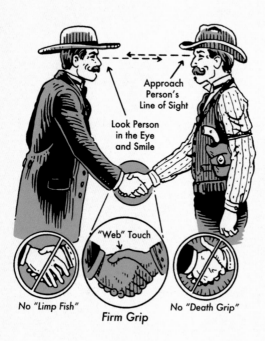

Approach Person's Line of Sight

Look Person in the Eye and Smile

"Web" Touch

No "Limp Fish"

Firm Grip

No "Death Grip"

— HOW —

1: MAKE sure your handshake is firm. Don't offer a limp fish grip, and don't crush the other person's hand with a death grip.

2: GO for the "web touch." You want the webbing between your thumb and index finger to meet the same spot on the other person's hand.

3: MAKE sure you don't have food or grease on your hands. The person you're meeting should remember you, not what you ate. Give sweaty hands a nonchalant wipe on your pants.

4: LOOK the person in the eye and smile.

WHEN

1: A good handshake requires good timing. At a party or social event, make sure to shake the host's hand when arriving and leaving. Shake hands with anyone you're meeting for the first time, as well as friends, family, and acquaintances with whom hugging doesn't seem appropriate.

2: SOME people avoid offering handshakes because they're afraid of being left hanging. If you're not sure if someone will notice your offer, extend your hand anyway. If you are left hanging, don't feel embarrassed. The problem isn't that the other person doesn't think you're important, but simply that your timing was off.

- Don't offer a handshake if the other person is engrossed in conversation with someone else.

- Don't approach someone from the side with your extended hand. It's hard to see.

- Audibly greet the person to get their attention and then offer your hand.

- Be aware of varying social norms. Most cultures have customs for when and if to shake hands.

WHERE

HANDSHAKES ARE good everywhere! Shake plenty of hands when you go to any social gathering, religious function (being sensitive to varying customs), family reunion, wedding, etc. Be liberal with your handshakes, and you'll perfect the art in no time.

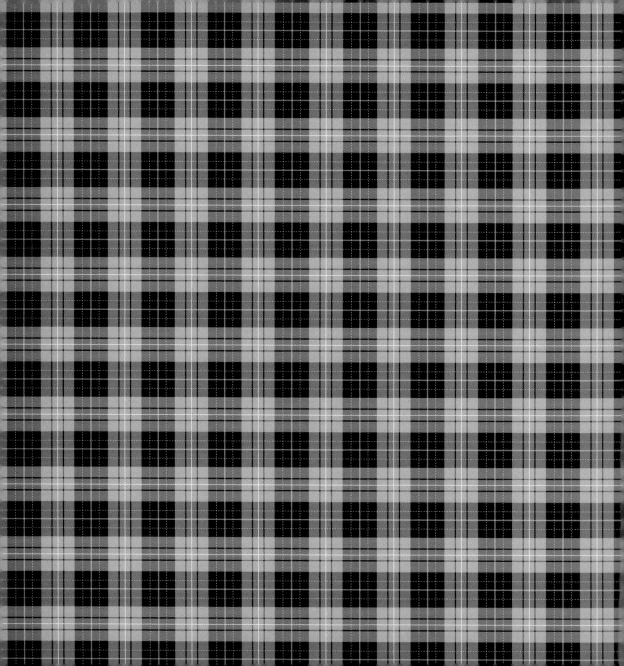

ACKNOWLEDGMENTS

Brett McKay

WHILE MY name is on the front cover of the book, there were a lot of people involved in making The Illustrated Art of Manliness a reality.

I'D FIRST like to thank Patrick Hutchison for the tremendous job in researching many of the illustrated guides that you found in this book. And thanks, Patrick, for being our go-to guy for illustrated guide content on artofmanliness.com.

THANK YOU to Jeremy Anderberg, our intrepid Jack-of-All-Trades at the Art of Manliness, for his work in managing the workflow process in the book and making sure that deadlines were met and details weren't overlooked. J, I appreciate all that you've done for the Art of Manliness these past four years.

THANK YOU to Ted Slampyak for his work on the book as well as for all the great work he's done for the Art of Manliness website over the years. Who would have known that an article about what it's like to be an illustrator would turn into such a fruitful partnership? Thanks, Ted!

THANKS TO our agents, Holly Root and Byrd Leavell at Waxman Leavell Literary Agency, for helping us get our book idea off the ground.

THANK YOU to our editor, Michael Szczerban, for his guidance and insight in helping shape its contents.

THANKS TO Mike Seeklander for his insights on how to disarm a gunman and a knifeman.

THANKS TO Greyfox Industries for their insights on how to protect your family like a VIP.

THANK YOU to Team O'Neil Rally School for allowing us to republish their article that they wrote for artofmanliness.com about recovering from car skids.

FINALLY, I'D like to thank my family. First, my kiddos, Gus and Scout. You two brighten my life. I'm so happy and proud that you're my children. I love you so much. Read this book. Both of you could learn a thing or two from it.

AND FINALLY, thank you to my wonderful wife, Kate. You're my Mate Woman and my partner in crime. I'm so blessed to have you in my life and that I get to work with you on the Art of Manliness. Thanks for all the amazing writing and editing you've done for the site over the years. You really know how to polish my writing turds into jewels. Thanks for the support and editing that you've provided on the book, too. I love you, always and forever.

Ted Slampyak

FIRST AND foremost, I want to thank my wife, Jennifer, for her support, feedback, and fantastic advice over the years of illustrating these guides. Her encouragement, love, and support have been and always will be essential. Thank you, my love.

OF COURSE I must thank Brett and Kate McKay for first having the idea of my illustrating some guides for their little site. They've turned out to be perfect partners, and good friends.

BRETT AND Jeremy Anderberg get my thanks for the writing, the research and reference, and the guidance that they've given me on every project. They always do the legwork that makes it easy for me to look good.

FURTHER READING

Chapter 1—The ADVENTURER

- *Norwegian Wood* by Lars Mytting
- *100 Deadly Skills: Survival Edition* by Clint Emerson
- *The Survivors Club* by Ben Sherwood
- *Survival Hacks* by Creek Stewart

Chapter 2—The GENTLEMAN

- *Modern Romance* by Aziz Ansari and Eric Klinenberg
- *Essential Manners for Men* by Peter Post
- *Esquire's Handbook for Hosts*

Chapter 3—The TECHNICIAN

- *Shop Class as Soulcraft* by Matthew Crawford
- *The Ax Book* by Dudley Cook
- *How Cars Work* by Tom Newton

Chapter 4—The WARRIOR

- *Starting Strength* by Mark Rippetoe
- *Solitary Fitness* by Charlie Bronson
- *Principles of Personal Defense* by Jeff Cooper

- *Left of Bang* by Patrick van Horne
- *100 Deadly Skills* by Clint Emerson

Chapter 5—The FAMILY MAN

- *Be Prepared: A Practical Handbook for New Dads* by Gary Greenberg
- *The Secrets of Happy Families* by Bruce Feiler
- *Couple Skills* by Patrick Fanning, Matthew McKay, and Kim Paleg
- *The Dangerous Book for Boys* by Conn and Hal Iggulden
- *The Happiest Baby on the Block* by Harvey Karp

Chapter 6—The LEADER

- *Science, Strategy and War* by Frans P. B. Osinga
- *The Charisma Myth* by Olivia Fox Cabane
- *Deskbound* by Kelly Starrett
- *How to Work a Room* by Susan RoAne

ABOUT THE ART OF MANLINESS

BRETT MCKAY founded The Art of Manliness in 2008 and has grown it into the largest independent men's interest magazine on the web. After graduating from the University of Oklahoma with a BA in Letters, he pursued his lifelong goal of going to law school. While attending the University of Tulsa College of Law, Brett started The Art of Manliness as something fun to do in his spare time. Brett and his wife, Kate, have two adorable children: Gus and Scout. Together they run AoM from its headquarters in Tulsa, OK.

TED SLAMPYAK is a freelance illustrator with over twenty years of professional experience in storyboards, comic strips and books, and spot illustrations for magazines, posters, and events. He has illustrated the bestselling book *100 Deadly Skills*, and his comics work includes six years on the long-running newspaper strip *Little Orphan Annie* as well as his own series, *Jazz Age*. Ted lives in Bernalillo, New Mexico, with his wife, designer and illustrator Jennifer Kinyak, and their two kids.

JEREMY ANDERBERG is the AoM jack-of-all-trades: editor, writer, podcast producer, and more. He went to Drake University in Des Moines, Iowa, and received degrees in both journalism and religious studies. Jeremy lives in the suburbs of Denver with his wife, Jane, and son, Graham.

PATRICK HUTCHISON was born and raised in the Pacific Northwest and has been writing about travel and the outdoors for over a decade. When not trying to fix the latest leak in his cabin's roof, he spends his time fishing, hiking, and fixing the latest leak in his boat.

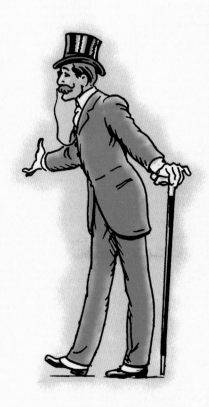